The Clinical & Medical Assessment

by

Merva Rivera

authorHOUSE™

1663 LIBERTY DRIVE, SUITE 200
BLOOMINGTON, INDIANA 47403
(800) 839-8640
WWW.AUTHORHOUSE.COM

First published by AuthorHouse 05/18/05

ISBN: 1-4184-1895-1 (e)
ISBN: 1-4184-1894-3 (sc)

Printed in the United States of America
Bloomington, Indiana

This book is printed on acid-free paper.

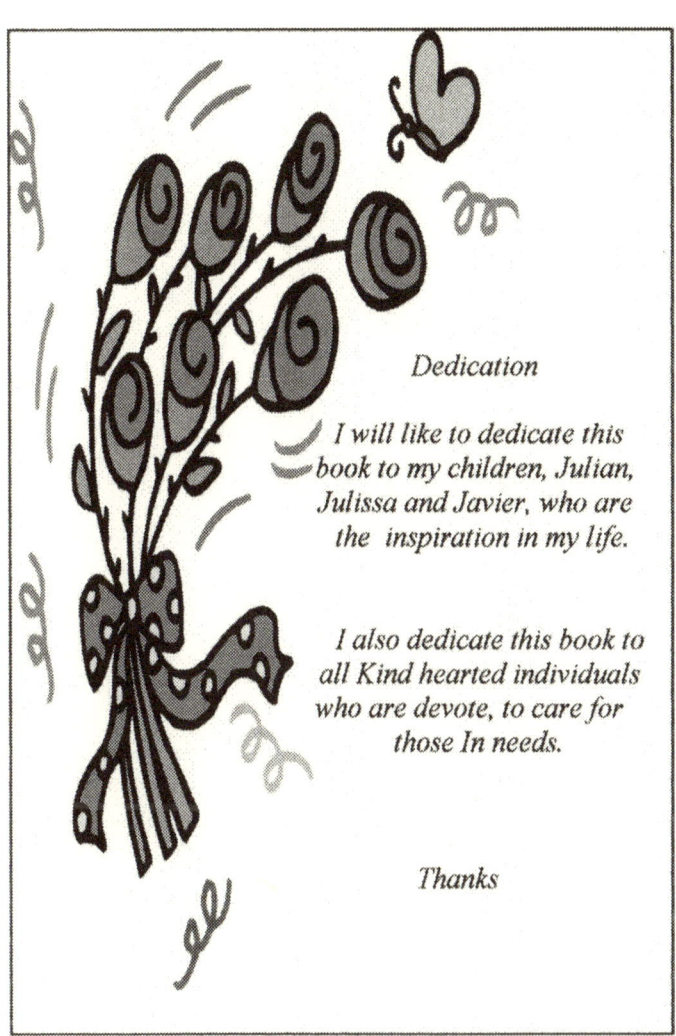

Dedication

*I will like to dedicate this
book to my children, Julian,
Julissa and Javier, who are
the inspiration in my life.*

*I also dedicate this book to
all Kind hearted individuals
who are devote, to care for
those In needs.*

Thanks

Respiration Range

Newborn	30-40
2 Year	25-32
4 Year	23-30
6 Year	21-26
8 Year	20-26
12 Year	18-22
16 Year	16-20
Adult	12-20

Note: **Stethoscope-** Device used to listen for organs sounds such as heart, lungs, bowels and arteries during blood pressure monitoring.

↑ **Tachypnea** / *fast*
* Nervous, Pain
* Exercise, fever
* Gas, Anxiety
* Decreased C02
* Shock, Ephedrine
* Lung disease e.g. (*COPD*)
* Cardiac disorder e.g. (*Heart failure*)
* Increased Carbon Dioxide
* Hemorrhage (*bleeding*)

Bradypnea /*slow* ↓
* Sleep
* Head Injury
* Morphine
* CVA (*stroke*)

Earpiece

Tubing

Diaphragm

Bell

Lungs sounds:
* *Wheeze: are high-pitched whistling sounds, caused by narrowing of the airway passageway.Example: Asthma*
* *Rales: make a Cracking or bubbling sound caused by air moving threw fluids. Example: Pulmonary Edema, & CHF.*
* *Ronchi: Low-pitched rumbling sounds resemble rales but Is continues like snoring. Example: Pneumonia.*

Merva Rivera

Pulse Reference

Pulse is the rhythmic expansion and contraction of an artery as blood is forced through it. An abnormal pulse rate may indicate sign of heart disorders or circulatory obstruction .e.g. a weak pulse may be caused by heart failure or shock. Characteristic of a pulse include: pulse rate which is the numbers of beats per minute, rhythm time between each pulse, volume refers to the strength of beat e.g. Strong, or weak and the condition of arterial wall this is asses when you palpate the skin.

Age	Average rate	Range
Birth	120	70 / 190
1 - 4 Years	120	80 /120
6-12 Years	90	70 /110
12-16 Years	75/ 90	60 /100
Adult	60/ 80	60 /100

↑Increased / *fast*　　　　Decreased / *Slow* ↓

Tachycardia
* Exertion
* Fright, Fever
* Hypertension
* Shock (*Hypovolemic*)
* Pain, infections

Bradycardia
* Cardiac problems
* Head injury
* Narcotics
* Some Poisons
* Mental depression
* Hypothyroidism

* Pulse deficit- is the different between apical rates and another pulse site rate.

* Pulse Pressure- is the different between the systolic and diastolic values. This formula is used to asses the Pressure In the arterial walls. A pulse pressure Over 50 points or under 30 is considered abnormal.

Example: 120 is systolic
　　　　- 100 is diastolic
　　　　20 pulse pressure

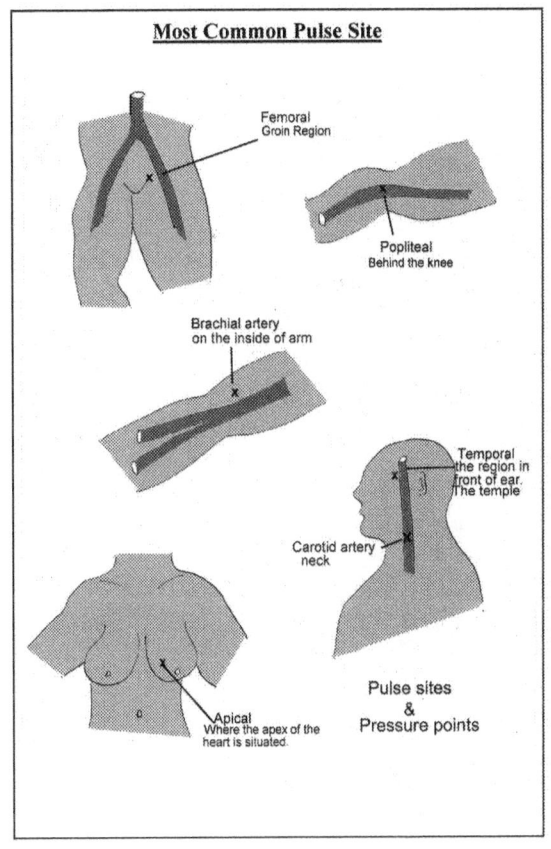

Most Common Pulse Site

Femoral
Groin Region

Popliteal
Behind the knee

Brachial artery
on the inside of arm

Temporal
the region in
front of ear.
The temple

Carotid artery
neck

Apical
Where the apex of the
heart is situated.

Pulse sites
&
Pressure points

BP / Blood Pressure value

High blood pressure is a lifelong diseases, it can be controlled but not cure. Management of high blood pressure includes low fat diets, low-salt diet, no smoking, moderate alcohol intake, losing weight, exercise and regular doctor check up. If persistent elevated blood pressure seeks medical advice for medication. Taking control of your pressure will lower the risk for emergencies such as strokes, heart attack and kidney failure. Another type of blood pressure is orthostatic (*postural*) hypotension is a sudden drop of blood pressure, an example: suddenly standing up, or may be causes by some medication. *Symptoms* include dizziness, blur vision or syncope.

Normal systolic ≤ **130** diastolic ≤ **85**
High Normal **130-139** diastolic **85-89**
≤Less Than ≥ Greater Than

Category	Systolic	Diastolic
Mild	140-159	90-99
High	160-179	100-109
Severe	180-209	110-119
Danger	≥ 209	≥ 119

Note: Right arm has a readings 3-4 mmhg(millimeter of mercury)
Higher than left arm. Sphygmomanometer- is a device used to measure BP.

Hypertension / high
↑ Increased BP
* Stress, Exercise
* High salt intake
* Head injury
* ASHD disease
* Renal, liver disease
* Smoking, obesity
* Hereditary

Hypotension / low
Decreased BP ↓
* Shock, Cancer
* Hemorrhage
* Infection, Fever
* Dehydration
* Weak heart
* Anemia

What is blood pressure? - It's the force of blood against the arteries. Systolic value represents the pressure created when the heart contracts. Diastolic represents relaxation and filling of the ventricles (lower heart chambers). Example:
Formula: 120 Systolic top numbers
                80 Diastolic bottom numbers

Reference for Pediatrics

Age	Systolic	Diastolic
Newborn	≤ 90	≤ 70mm hg
1-5 years	≤100	≤ 70
Older -9	≤120	≤ 84
Older-13	100 + age = systolic Diastolic is 30-40 beats less than systolic	

Apgar scoring --A system used to evaluate a Newborn Physical condition after birth, its scores at 1 minute after birth and 5 minutes later for a total not to exceed 10. Scores: 0-3 indicates distress, 4-6 modern distresses, and 7-10 is mild.

Apgar scoring

Sign	0	1 points	2 points
Heart Rate	Absent	Below 100	Over 100
Respiration Rate	Absent	Slow / Irregular	Normal crying
Muscle tone	Limp	Some flexion extremities	Active; good motion in extremities
Irritability	No response	Crying: grimace	Crying, cough, or sneeze
Skin color	Blue or Paleness	Pink / blue extremities	Pink the entire body

<u>Temperature</u>

Temperature is controlled by the Hypothalamus an area in the brain that acts as a thermostat. Normal body temperature is 98.6° however it varies during the day. Most common factors affecting temperatures are, exercise, sleep, infections, weather or illness. Elevated temperature is called a fever or medically known as *Pyrexia* ,this condition is most often the cause for seizures in young children's. Fever it's commonly triggered by a bacterial or virus infections.

Site	Color tip	Time
Oral	Blue	3 Minutes
Rectal	Red	3-5 Minutes
Axillary	Silver	15 Minutes

Normal Values reference

Oral (*By mouth*) under tongue	98.6 ° F	37 ° c
Rectal Method –Most accurate reading, recommended for children under the age of 6 & unconscious patients. Lubricate and insert 1-1½ inch or tip.	99.6 ° F	36.4 ° c
Axillary (*under armpits*)	97.6 ° F	36.4°c
Tympanic (*via Ear*)	98.6 ° F	37 ° c

Fahrenheit to Celsius
(F°) – 32 x by 0.555
Example:
95.0 (F°) - 32 = 63
63 x   0.555 = 34.965
Round off   35.0 C°

Celsius to Fahrenheit
(C°) X 1.8 then add 32
Example:
35 C° x 1.8 = 63.0
63.0 + 32 = 95 F°

Multiplication Table

1	2	3	4	5	6	7	8	9	10
2	4	6	8	10	12	14	16	18	20
3	6	9	12	15	18	21	24	27	30
4	8	12	16	20	24	28	32	36	40
5	10	15	20	25	30	35	40	45	50
6	12	18	24	30	36	42	48	54	60
7	14	21	28	35	42	49	56	63	70
8	16	24	32	40	48	56	64	72	80
9	18	27	36	45	54	63	72	81	90
10	20	30	40	50	60	70	80	90	100

Kilogram to lbs

Kilogram   X   2.2 = Lbs
1 Kilogram = 2.2 pound
Example:
68 Kilogram x 2.2 = 149.6 lbs

Pound to Kilogram

Lbs x 0.45 = kg
1 lbs = 0.45 Kg
Example:
120 lbs x 0.45 = 54 kg

Drugs Calculations

Formula:
Dose ordered = Amount administered
Dose available

Example: Tablets $\frac{15\ mg}{5\ mg}$ = 3 Tablets

Example: Liquid $\frac{35\ mg}{50\ mg/ml}$ = 0.7 ml

Solution Concentration
Formula:
$\frac{Dosage\ in\ solution}{Volume\ of\ solution}$ = Solution concentration

Example: $\frac{100\ mg}{500\ ml}$ = 0.2mg/ml

IV Dose Rate Calculation
Formula:
$\frac{Dose\ Ordered}{Solution\ concentration}$ = Volume/ Hour

Example: $\frac{50\ mg/hr}{2\ mg/ml}$ = 25 ml/hr

The Eye & disorders

Is the organ of sight, it consists of structures that focus an image onto the retina. The retina is a membrane that lined the back of the eyes, it contains specialized nerves cells that convert light energy into nerves impulses and transmit via the optic nerve the image to the brain where is recorded and interpreter.

Pupil's Assessments

Dilated, Unresponsive	Cardiac arrest, Drugs such as: LSD, amphetamines.
Constricted, Unresponsive	Central nervous disease, Narcotic such as: heroin, morphine, or codeine
Unequal	Stroke, head injury
Lackluster, Pupils don't focus	Shock, coma

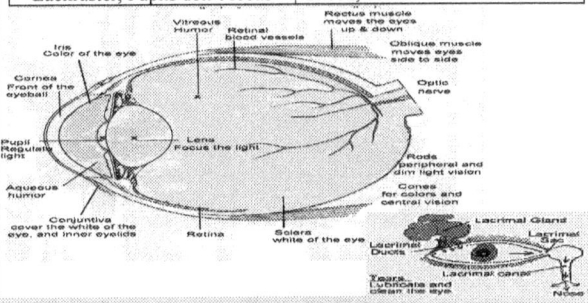

Most Common Conditions of the eyes

* **Hyperopia**-*(farsightedness)* is when the eye is too short from front to back, near objects becomes blur, because the lights ray meet beyond the retina, recommended treatment is the use of convex lenses to reinforce focusing power.
* **Myopia**- *(Nearsightedness)* is when the eye is too long from front t to back, far away objects looks blur because the light rays entering the eye meet in front of the retina instead on it, recommended treatment use of Concave lens.
* **Cataract**-when the lens of the eye becomes cloudy, it prevents light entering the eye and distorts vision ,causes may be due to disease or often the aging process.
* **Astigmatism**- caused by a variation of shape and focusing of the eye.
* **Glaucoma**- A condition in which the pressure of fluid in the eye is too high.
* **Color blindness**- occurs when cones in the eyes are insufficient. Colors most commonly affected are Red, green and blue.

The Human Ear

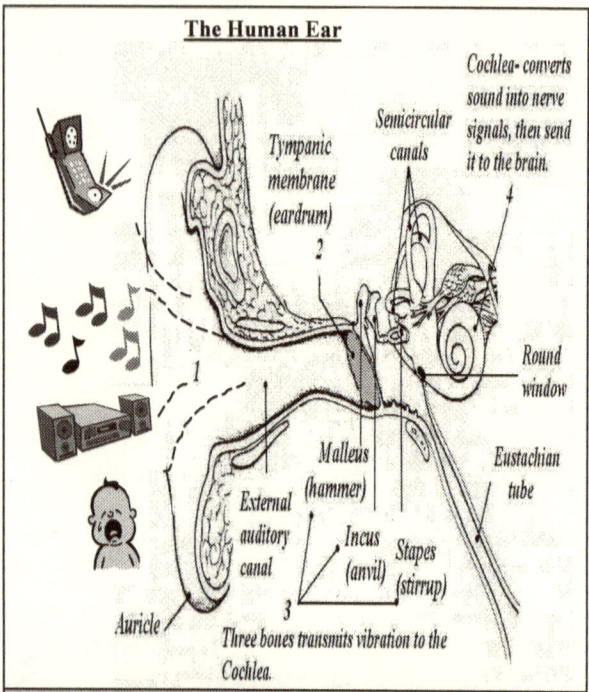

Cochlea- converts sound into nerve signals, then send it to the brain.

Semicircular canals

Tympanic membrane (eardrum)

2

4

Round window

Malleus (hammer)

Eustachian tube

External auditory canal

Incus (anvil)

Stapes (stirrup)

1

3

Auricle

Three bones transmits vibration to the Cochlea.

The human Ear: The ear and the brain provide your sense of hearing. The ear converts sound waves into electrical nerves impulses, and then it send to the brain for interpretation. The ear is divide into three parts, the outer that is the visible portion which collects and funnel sound wave into the ear. The middle ear contains the bones which vibrates sounds and send it into the inner ear which is beyond the cochlea a *(shell like shape)* structures and the canals, then its send impulses to the nerves and finally the brain. The ears also contain specialized glands called the *Cerumen* located in the external canals; it produces a waxy substance that traps dust and dirt and prevent it from entering.

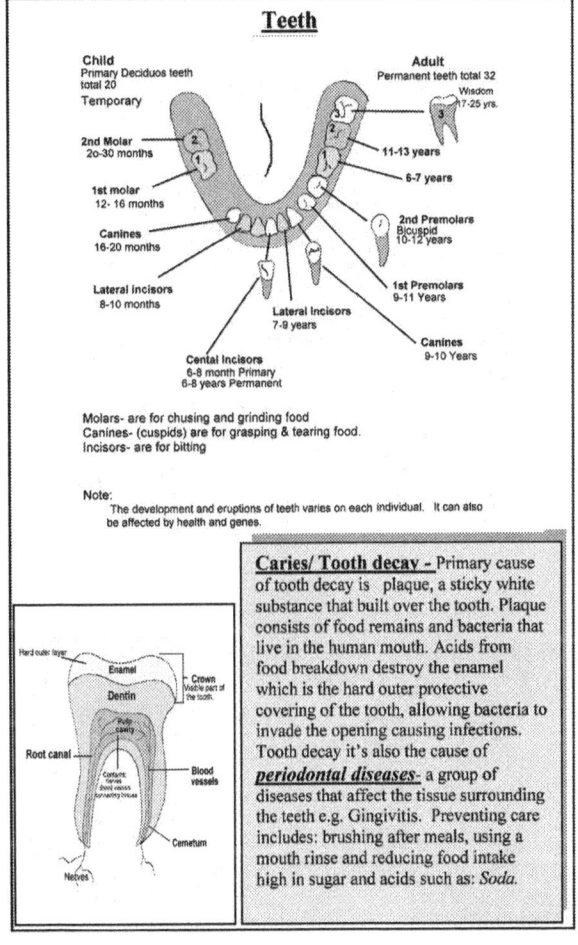

Teeth

Child
Primary Deciduos teeth total 20
Temporary

Adult
Permanent teeth total 32
Wisdom 17-25 yrs.

2nd Molar 2o-30 months

1st molar 12-16 months

Canines 16-20 months

Lateral incisors 8-10 months

Cental Incisors
6-8 month Primary
6-8 years Permanent

Lateral Incisors 7-9 years

11-13 years

6-7 years

2nd Premolars Bicuspid 10-12 years

1st Premolars 9-11 Years

Canines 9-10 Years

Molars- are for chusing and grinding food
Canines- (cuspids) are for grasping & tearing food.
Incisors- are for bitting

Note:
The development and eruptions of teeth varies on each individual. It can also be affected by health and genes.

Hard outer layer
Enamel
Dentin
Crown Visible part of the tooth.
Pulp cavity
Root canal
Contains nerves, blood vessels & connecting tissues
Blood vessels
Cementum
Nerves

Caries/ Tooth decay - Primary cause of tooth decay is plaque, a sticky white substance that built over the tooth. Plaque consists of food remains and bacteria that live in the human mouth. Acids from food breakdown destroy the enamel which is the hard outer protective covering of the tooth, allowing bacteria to invade the opening causing infections. Tooth decay it's also the cause of *periodontal diseases*- a group of diseases that affect the tissue surrounding the teeth e.g. Gingivitis. Preventing care includes: brushing after meals, using a mouth rinse and reducing food intake high in sugar and acids such as: *Soda.*

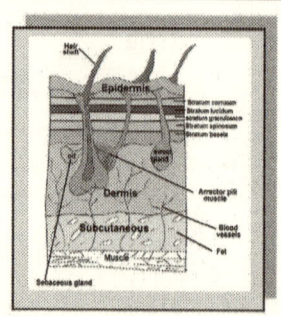

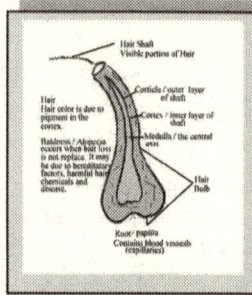

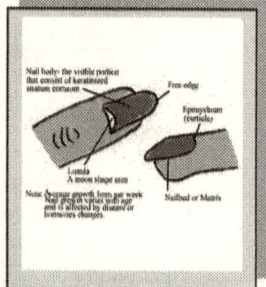

Skin assessments -Skin is an important indicator of health because many disorders can cause skin color changes. Skin evaluation consists of, rash, lesions, bruise and color.

Skin color	Possible cause
Red / Hot	Stroke, alcohol, Heart attack, infections, High blood pressure, blushing, or infectious disease.
White / cold	Shock, anemia, heart attack, Fright, & fainting
Blue	Asphyxia (*suffocation*), hypoxia (*Lack of oxygen*), heart attack, poisoning.
Yellow	Liver disease (*Hepatitis*) & Gallbladder
Black & Blue	Blood Under the skin

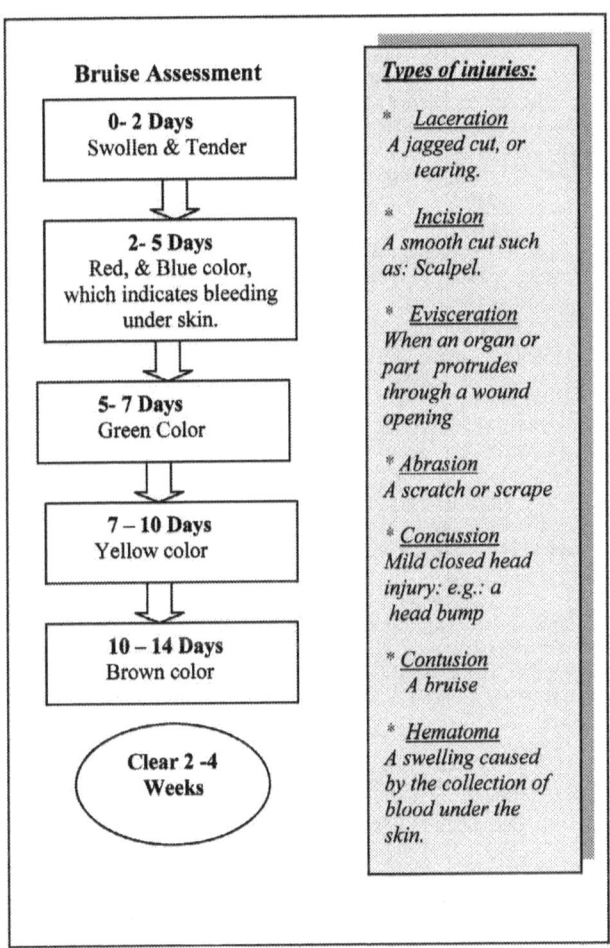

Bruise Assessment

0- 2 Days
Swollen & Tender

2- 5 Days
Red, & Blue color,
which indicates bleeding
under skin.

5- 7 Days
Green Color

7 – 10 Days
Yellow color

10 – 14 Days
Brown color

Clear 2 -4
Weeks

Types of injuries:

* *Laceration*
*A jagged cut, or
tearing.*

* *Incision*
*A smooth cut such
as: Scalpel.*

* *Evisceration*
*When an organ or
part protrudes
through a wound
opening*

* *Abrasion*
A scratch or scrape

* *Concussion*
*Mild closed head
injury: e.g.: a
head bump*

* *Contusion*
A bruise

* *Hematoma*
*A swelling caused
by the collection of
blood under the
skin.*

Bleeding

External bleeding is visible blood loss. Internal bleeding is within; causes can be medical as in ulcers or traumatic. Most common signs & symptoms for internal bleeding are: bruise or contusion on site, pain, vomiting or coughing blood and stool that are black or bright Red.

First aid for Bleeding

Do's	&	Don't
Direct pressure Apply Direct pressure with sterile dressing over wound to slow down bleeding. Approximately time (*10-30*) minutes.		**Do Not** Removed soak dressings because it will reactivate bleeding; apply another dressing on top if needed.
Elevation Using gravity Elevate if possible while applying pressure to slow down blood flow.		**Do Not** Elevates if suspected fracture or if impale object. Never removed a penetrating object.
Pressure Point Applied pressure at nearest artery If bleeding continues.		**Pressure points** Brachial artery for arm. Femoral for lower limbs. Temporal for scalp.
Tourniquet This method is used at a last resort and with extreme caution. Tourniquet should be 3-4 inches wide, tie above a joint.		**Do Not** Loosen, it may released clot or toxic into blood stream. Make note of time applied; it may prevent the lost of a limb.

Types of bleeding:
- **Arterial bleeding-** is high-pressure, oxygenated blood, flow is fast, profuse & bright red color.
- **Venous Bleeding-** is low pressure deoxygenated blood, Steady flow and dark color.
- **Capillary bleeding-** Blood oozes, this type of injury often clots and stops by itself e.g. *paper cut.*

Decubitus Ulcers

Also commonly refers as Bedsores, pressure sores and decubitus, it's caused by the breakdown of the skin due to frictions, and prolonged pressures e.g.:

  *. *Laying in one position for too long or wearing a cast.*
  * *Poor circulation / Insufficient blood flow that brings cell nourishment.*

Decubitus ulcers occur most frequently where the bone lies close to the skin surface. These are often called pressure sores since they bear the body weight when the patient is sitting or lying down.

Decubitus are most common in patients who are:
- Elderly, Very thin
- Obese (*overweight*)
- Unable to move e.g. *(paralyzed)*
- Incontinent

Most common site includes:
- Toes, heels, ankle and knee
- Elbow and shoulder blade
- Spine (*Tail bone area*)
- Back of the head and over ears

These sites are for sores often-found in obese patients:
- Under breasts, between buttock
- Between the thighs

Treatment may include:
- Keep broken skin covered
- Maintain skin dry and clean
- Remove pressure from area
- Massage skin surrounding to increase blood flow

The stages of skin breakdown

Skin breakdown occurs in four stages.

Stage 1	Redness and hot skin
Stage 2	Skin is red with blister like lesions or skin is broken
Stage 3	All layers of the skin are broken, deep crater has formed, High risk of infections.
Stage 4	The ulcer has eroded skin and other tissues are damage muscle and bone can be visible. Foul rotten odor

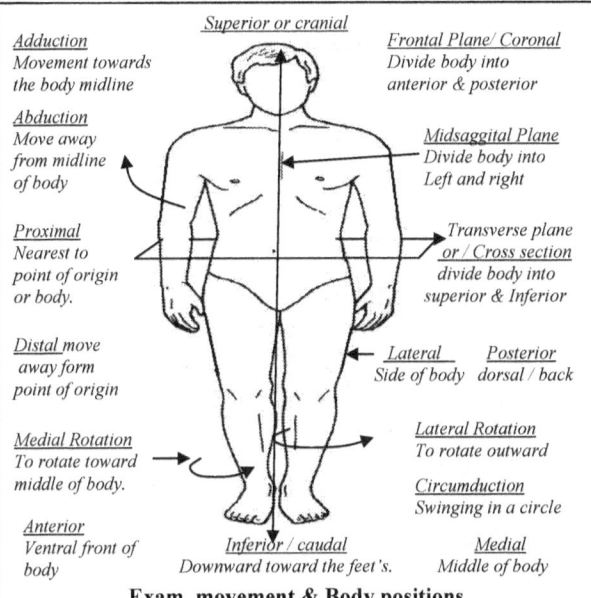

Superior or cranial

Adduction
Movement towards
the body midline

Abduction
Move away
from midline
of body

Proximal
Nearest to
point of origin
or body.

Distal move
away form
point of origin

Medial Rotation
To rotate toward
middle of body.

Anterior
Ventral front of
body

Frontal Plane/ Coronal
Divide body into
anterior & posterior

Midsaggital Plane
Divide body into
Left and right

Transverse plane
or / Cross section
divide body into
superior & Inferior

Lateral   Posterior
Side of body dorsal / back

Lateral Rotation
To rotate outward

Circumduction
Swinging in a circle

Inferior / caudal
Downward toward the feet's.

Medial
Middle of body

Exam, movement & Body positions

Anatomical Position- is standing erect, face forward, arms on the sides, with palm and toes forward.	**Trendelenberg-** also known as the shock positions, may also be use for fainting victim. Feet's are elevated 12" above head, which increases blood and oxygen to the brain and upper organs.
Prone- *(laying Ventral)* face down on stomach. Position used to exam back and spine.	
Sim's or **Lateral-** is laying patient on side of the body, for recovery, enemas and rectal examination.	**Fowler's** – sitting upright with head elevate at 90° angle degree, position use to examine head, chest, and neck of for feeding. **Semi Fowler's** is angle at 45°.
Supine- patients *(Laying Dorsal)* on back, face up, for an abdomen, breast or frontal examination.	

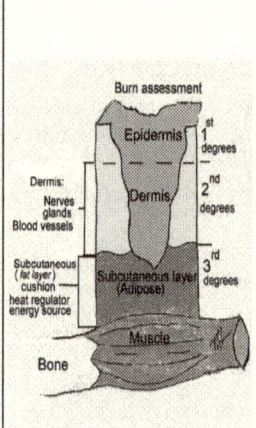

1st degree (*Superficial*) affects the epidermis, which is the outer layer of the skin. Example: Sun burn.

Signs & symptoms:
- Redness, mild swelling
- Tenderness and pain

Tx: *Apply cold usually 10 –20 minutes to stop the internal burning, use a skin moisturizer to prevent dryness or Aloe vera, which has an Antimicrobial agent and an analgesic effect.*

2nd degree (*Partial Thickness*) destroyed the Epidermis (*Outer skin*) and Dermis (*Inner*) layer of the skin.

Signs &symptoms:
- Blister, swelling,
- Weeping of fluid, and painful

Tx: *Cool with cold compress and cover with sterile dressing to prevent infections and never break blisters.*

3rd degree *(Full thickness)* is severe burn that destroys all three-skin layers, deep into muscle and bone. Skin graft is needed.

Signs & Symptoms:
- Dry skin, charred or white
- No pain, nerves are affected

Tx: *seek Immediate Medical attention, high risk of dehydration and infections.*

Types of Burns:

Thermal- Caused by hot liquids, Vapors, radiation or Flames.

Electrical- AC or DC currents (*high or low voltage of electricity*), or lightning.

Radiation- Caused by ultraviolet ray (*Sunburn*) or an atomic explosion.

Chemical- Caused by wet or dry corrosive substances that come in contact with the skin such as: acids, alkalis and organic compound.

Burn assessments

Adult — 9 head

18 Front   Rule of 9

9   9

18 Back

18   18

Infant

Body parts	value
Head	18
Front	18
Back	18
L.arm	9
R.arm	9
L.Leg	14
R.leg	14
Genital	1

*When considering the severity of burn, consider the following factors: **agent or source**, **body region** consider the location and other organs, **Degree of burn**, degree of burn can be assess using the rule of 9 method to approximately estimate the extent of burn, **age** of the patient and finally the past **medical history** of a patient which can complicated matters.*

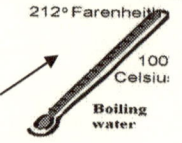

Heat Emergencies

Heat Cramps- Sudden Painful muscle cramp usually occurs in the leg and abdomen, caused by mild dehydration due to profuse sweating and loss of electrolytes.
Most common Signs & Symptoms: Dizziness, exhaustion, or faint.

Heat Exhaustion- Is a severe loss of fluids due to excessive heat exposure. Most common in the summer, among firefighter, and poor ventilated apartment. It can lead to Heatstroke a life-threatening emergency. Patients may feel weak, severe thirst, nausea, dizziness, headache, abdominal cramps, and possible unconsciousness.

Heat Stroke - It's a type of Shock. This condition is when the body temperature reaches above 107° degrees; it becomes dehydrated causing organs failure or death. Patient may present dilated pupils, seizures, loss of consciousness and possible coma.

Heat Exposure Emergencies

Condition	Breathing	Pulse	Skin
Cramps	Varies	Varies	Moist Warm
Heat Exhaustion	Rapid / shallow	Weak	Cold Clammy
Heat stroke	Deep then Shallow	Full rapid	Dry-hot

First Aid for mild case of heat exhaustion:
- Remove Victim from heat source
- Begin cooling process, raise legs
- Replace fluid loss e.g. Water.

Excessive Cold

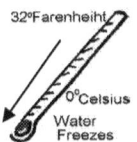

32°Farenheiht

0°Celsius
Water
Freezes

Hypothermia- it's a Life threatening Emergency where the body temperature falls below the normal 98.6°, most common causes are exposure to excessive cold, such as winds, winter and freezing waters. Be aware that exposure to cold often lead to dehydration.

Most common signs & symptoms:

- Shivering, slurred speech, cyanosis *(Blue)*
- Frostbite in the ear, nose, fingers, hand ect.
- Shallow, low breathing and faint pulse
- Lethargy, Unconsciousness
- Coma with dilated and fixed pupils
- Cold pale skin

Frostnip- *(Frosting)* - Is the First stage of frostbite, caused by prolonged exposure to cold. The skin becomes red or white and numb. It often affects expose body parts, for *example:* the face, hand, ears and nose.

Frostbite- Is the Second stages of freezing, deep frostbite causes Ice crystal in the skin and deep into the subcutaneous layers, it also affect body structure within such as: Muscle, bone, blood vessels, and organs can become frozen. If not treated it can lead to gangrene and lost of limbs.

Condition	Skin surface	Tissue under	Skin color
Frostnip	Soft	Soft	Red & White
Frostbite	Hard	Soft	White & waxy
Freezing	Hard	Hard	Blotchy white gray to blue

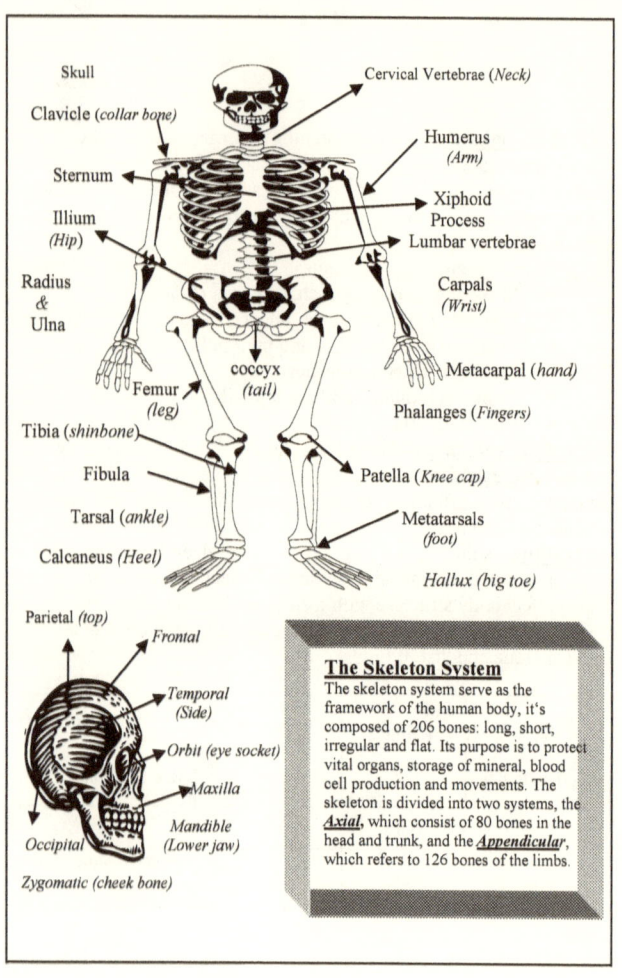

Skull

Cervical Vertebrae (*Neck*)

Clavicle (*collar bone*)

Humerus
(*Arm*)

Sternum

Xiphoid
Process

Illium
(*Hip*)

Lumbar vertebrae

Radius
&
Ulna

Carpals
(*Wrist*)

coccyx
(*tail*)

Femur
(*leg*)

Metacarpal (*hand*)

Phalanges (*Fingers*)

Tibia (*shinbone*)

Fibula

Patella (*Knee cap*)

Tarsal (*ankle*)

Metatarsals
(*foot*)

Calcaneus (*Heel*)

Hallux (*big toe*)

Parietal *(top)*

Frontal

Temporal
(*Side*)

Orbit (*eye socket*)

Maxilla

Mandible
(*Lower jaw*)

Occipital

Zygomatic (*cheek bone*)

The Skeleton System

The skeleton system serve as the framework of the human body, it's composed of 206 bones: long, short, irregular and flat. Its purpose is to protect vital organs, storage of mineral, blood cell production and movements. The skeleton is divided into two systems, the **_Axial_**, which consist of 80 bones in the head and trunk, and the **_Appendicular_**, which refers to 126 bones of the limbs.

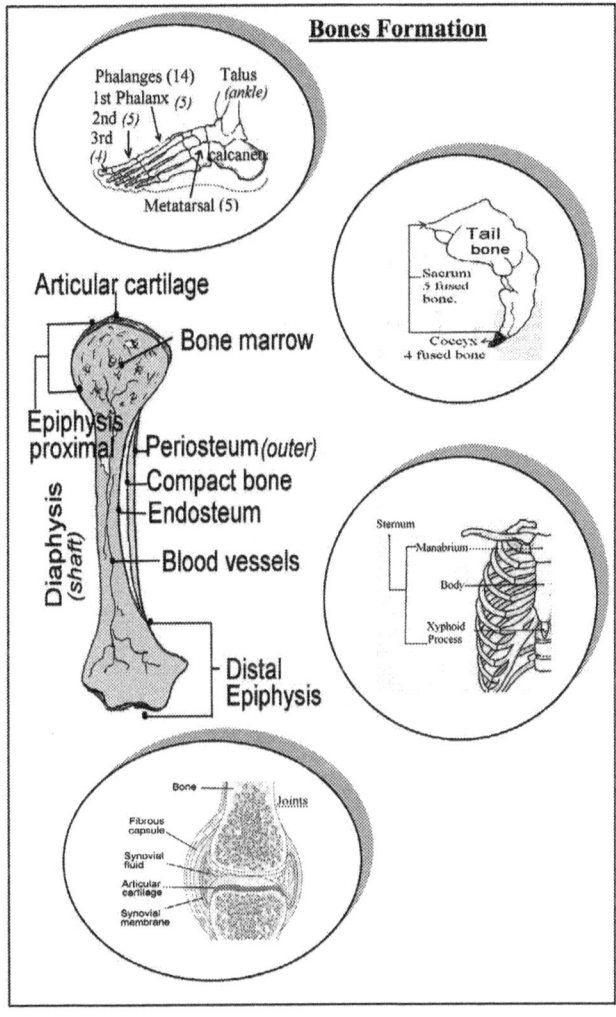

Bones Formation

Phalanges (14)   Talus *(ankle)*
1st Phalanx *(5)*
2nd *(5)*
3rd *(4)*   calcaneu
Metatarsal (5)

Tail bone
Sacrum
5 Fused bone.
Coccyx
4 fused bone

Articular cartilage
Bone marrow
Epiphysis proximal
Periosteum *(outer)*
Compact bone
Endosteum
Diaphysis *(shaft)*
Blood vessels
Distal Epiphysis

Sternum
Manubrium
Body
Xyphoid Process

Bone   Joints
Fibrous capsule
Synovial fluid
Articular cartilage
Synovial membrane

 Joints- or Articulation is where two bones connect; it's composed of fibrous connective tissue, and cartilage. Joints are classified into three categories: *Synarthroses* immovable ,*Amphiarthroses* slightly movable and *Diarthroses* freely movable joints. Movable Joints are encased in a tough fibrous capsule, lined with a synovial membrane that secrets a sticky, clear, fluids call the *synovial*, which lubricate the joints. In certain type of arthritis the synovial membrane becomes inflamed and the fluid becomes viscous, this act reduces lubrication and the increase of friction and movement becomes difficult and painful. Most common joint disorders are dislocation out of place, arthritis and Bursitis. Joints produce different movement, for example:

* **Ball & socket**- permits widest range of motion such as backward, forward and rotation e.g. shoulder & hip.
* **Condyloid**-Angular motion not rotation: Metacarpals
* **Saddle**-permits wide range of movement such as side to side and back and forth *e.g.* found in thumb.
* **Pivot**-limited rotation-*e.g.* joint between atlas and axis located in the spine.
* **Hinge**-allows flexion and extension *e.g.* knee &, elbow
* **Gliding**-sliding or twisting *e.g.* between carpals & tarsal.

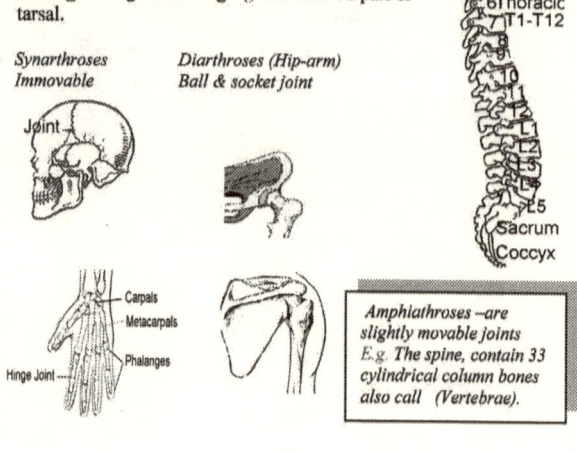

Synarthroses
Immovable

Diarthroses (Hip-arm)
Ball & socket joint

Amphiathroses –are slightly movable joints E.g. The spine, contain 33 cylindrical column bones also call (Vertebrae).

Fractures

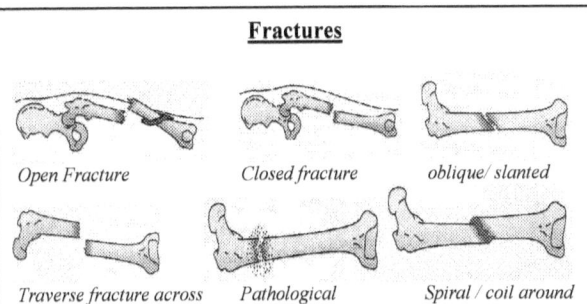

Open Fracture *Closed fracture* *oblique/ slanted*

Traverse fracture across *Pathological* *Spiral / coil around*

Bones are composed mostly of mineral such as calcium and phosphorus which make it hard. The central cavity contains the bone marrow in which blood cells are produced. A fracture is a break in the bone, it may be the result from an injury caused by Direct force on the bone, Indirect force where injury occur in another site or pathological, which is caused by diseases such as *Osteoporosis*. Open Fracture is a broken expose bone, with skin damage & bleeding. Closed fracture is an internal break, without skin injury. *Note: Crepitus-* is the grating sound heard when two bones rub together most common in fractures.

Sprain	Strain	Dislocations
Ligaments- are strong band of connecting tissue which Connect bone to bone. A Sprain is a torn ligament, Most common in the Knee & ankles due to sudden twisting or weight.	*Tendons -* Is a fibrous connecting tissue which Connect bone to muscle. A strain is a torn or overstretches muscle. Most common in the lower back due to improper lifting or in overstretch exercise.	*A joint-* is where two bone meet. Dislocation Occurs when bones are pull apart from it normal position in a joint. Most common site is: the Elbow, knee, fingers, shoulder, ankles, or hip. *Complication :* Many blood vessel and nerves can be affected if injured.
S/S : Swelling Discoloration Pain on movement	*S/S:* Pain	*S/S:* Deformity Swelling Pain Loss of motion.

First aid
For
Soft tissue injuries

R - **Rest**

> *Rest injured part, and avoid any pressure or weight on site. Injuries heal faster if rested.*

I - **Ice**

> *Apply Ice pack for 20-30 minutes, Caution: not to freeze body part. Ice helps reduced swelling by constricting blood vessels and it also reduces pain.*

C - **Compression**

> *Compression reduced swelling. Applied an ace bandage to immobilized site, Caution do not constrict circulation.*

E - **Elevation**

> *Elevation help decreased swelling.*

Note:
Heat application- has the opposite effect than cold, it dilate blood vessels, increased blood circulation and oxygen. Heat Stimulation help tissues heal faster for example: a sprains or muscle injuries. Heat should not be used until after 48 hour of injury, this method is also helpful for bruise.

Venipucture
Recommended 21 –22 gauge
Applied Tourniquet 3-4 inches above elbow

Most common site used is the antecubital area. After blood collection invert tube 8-10 times.

Tube color	Additive
Yellow	Sodium SPS
Marble	Gel / SST
Blue	Sodium Citrate
Green	Heparin
Purple/ lavender	EDTA
Gray	Potassium Oxalate Fluoride

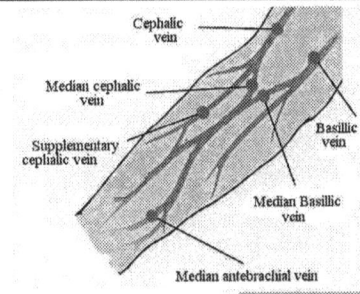

Types of Blood Vessels

Arteries- are located deep, have muscular thicker walls and a pulse.

Veins- are superficial, bouncing when touch and have valves to prevent blood back up, no pulse.

Capillaries- are Microscopic vessels, where oxygen and carbon dioxide are exchanged.

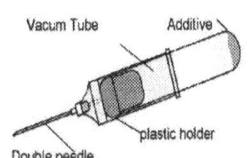

Most Common Blood Test & Tubes

Red Marble / speckle SST tube
Cardiac, thyroid, Comprehensive metabolic panels, Basic metabolic panels, Bun (*blood urea nitrogen*), Albumin, HDL, FSH, LH, GGT, cholesterol, Renal and liver function, hepatitis panel, HIV test, lipid panels, LDL/HDL, measles mumps, Rubella IgG, varicella, electrolyte, Potassium, SGPT, SGOT,THS/ high sensitive, RPR, syphilis.

Lavender / Purple Tube
Additives; Ethylenediamine tetraacetic acid
Most common Test:
ABO and RH, CBC & Platelets, Hemoglobin (*Hgb*),Hematocrits(*Hct*), Platelets , Sed rate, thrombocytes,mono-spot, RBC/WBC HgbAIC, sickle cell screen test.

Blue top tube
Additives: *Sodium Citrate*
Most commonTest:
PT/ PTT, B-hCG, Thrombin T, Fibrinogen Lupus anticoag, Factor Assay, D-DIMER Antithromb3, Coumadin, Heparin.

Green Top tube
Additives :Heparin
Most commonTest:
Lead screening
Gray Tube *(Potassium oxalate)*
Test:
GTT/Glucose Tolerance, Alcohol

Centrifuge
Laboratory machine used to separate cells and other elements in the blood.

Vacuun tube
Timer
Power

Hct **Hematocrit Value** %

It's the value of erythrocytes in a given percentage

Neonate	44-64
1 Month	35-49
6 Month	30-40
1-10 years	35-41
Men	42-52
Women	36-45

Hgb **Hemoglobin Reference**

It's the iron pigment found in Red blood cells, its primary function is to carry oxygen from the lungs to the tissues.

Neonate	17-23
Infant	9- 14
Adult female	12-16
Adult Male	15-18

The Average adult has about 10 pints of Blood (*5- 6 Quarts*). Blood carries nutrients, oxygen, antibodies, hormones and eliminates wastes product such as carbon dioxide. Blood is composed of 55% plasma which consists of mostly water and substance such as proteins; fats, glucose and salt, 45% of blood are formed elements which are the cells bodies such as:

- RBC-also called red blood cell or (*Erythrocytes*) function is to transports oxygen. RBC has a life span of 120 days before Hemolysis that is the destruction of cells, when breakdown occurs hemoglobin is release into the blood for new cells. Premature breakdown leads to anemia and Jaundice.
  WBC- White cells (Leukocytes) protect the body from infections by creating antibodies and effulging bacteria.
  Thrombocytes-Platelets (*clotting*) stop bleeding by clotting.

→ 55 % Plasma (*clear liquid after cell separation/ Centrifuge*)

→ 45% Formed elements (*the cells)*

Blood Cells & Type

Blood cells are formed within the bone marrow. There are three types: RBC's also called Erythrocytes, the production of RBC's are influence by a hormone produced in the kidney called Erythropoietin. , RBC's are most numerous; they have a biconcave disc shape and no nucleus. WBC's also called Leukocytes, are the largest, it's divides into two categories: 1- **_Granulocytes_** –it contains a granules cytoplasm and may have an oddly shaped nucleus, there are three of this types: *Neutrophils, eosinophils*, and *basophils*. 2- **_Agranulocytes-_** they have few granules in cytoplasm, two types are: *Monocytes* also called Macrophage and *Lymphocyte*. Elevation of Leukocytes is called Leukocytosis, possible causes include: infections, leukemia, appendicitis, and pneumonia. A decreased in leukocyte is called Leukopenia, possible causes are: exposure to radiation, certain chemicals and drugs. Platelets are responsible for clotting and stop bleeding.

Average blood count

Cells	Neonate	children	Adult male	Adult female
RBC millions	4.8 – 7.1 million	4.5- 4.8 million	4.5- 6.0 million	4.0-5.5 million
WBC thousands	9,000- to- 30,000	5,000 –to- 13,000	4,000 -11,000	
Platelets Hundred thousands	140,000 -to- 300,000	150,000 – 450,000	150,000 – 400,000	

The term Blood type refers to the antigen present in the Red Blood cell membrane. An antigen is a substance that causes the formation of antibodies. Proper blood type is very important because formation of antibodies can cause the red blood cell of a donor to become clumped and rejected if not compatible. Type O is considered universal blood type, because blood can be given to anyone. Type AB is considered universal recipients, because they can receive blood from most donors. The Rh (*Rhesus*) antigen is either positive or negative; a person must receive the same Rh factor from a donor to be compatible, this type is of great concern in pregnancy when mother and unborn are opposite it can lead to complication or even death.

Blood typing

Type	Red Blood cell antigen	Donate to	Received from
A	A	A, AB	A,O
B	B	AB, B	B,O
AB	AB	AB	A,B,AB,O
O	None	A,B,AB,O	O

Cholesterol value

Cholesterol is a lipid found in saturated fat, it's also produced in the body, Its' function are source of energy, carries fat soluble vitamin A & D, and supplies fatty acids for growth.

Good fats is known as HDL high-density lipoprotein and are found in diets containing Polysaturated or monounsaturated fat. Bad fat are known as LDL low density lipoprotein found in cholesterol and saturated fats.

≤ Less than ≥ Greater than

HDL 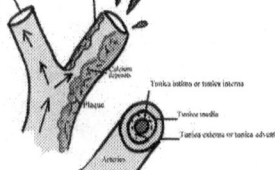	Desirable	≥ 35mg/dl
LDL	Desirable	>130mg/dl
	Border	130- 159mg/dl
	High risk	≥160 mg/dl
Cholesterol		
Desirable		< 200mg/dl
Border high		200-239 mg/dl
High risk		≥240 mg/dl
Triglycerides		
Desirable		< 250 mg/dl

The walls of an arteries consists three layers:
* Tunica externa consists of Connective tissue.
* Tunica media is primary smooth muscle and is the thickest.
* Tunica interna consists of simple squamous epithelium.

Urine Reference	
Color	Clear / Amber
Gravity	1.001-1.035
PH	4.6-8.0
Protein (mg/dl)	Negative
Glucose/dl)	Negative
Ketone (mg/dl)	Negative
BilirubinUA	Negative
Blood	Negative
Nitrite (mg/dl)	Negative
Urobilinogen	0.1-1.0
WBC	Negative

<u>Kidney</u>-Red brown bean shaped granular organs, Located in the Retroperitoneal Region. The Kidneys are responsible for filtering the blood and eliminating waste from the body such as breakdown of protein and excess water, it also controls body acid-base balance and it produces some hormones.

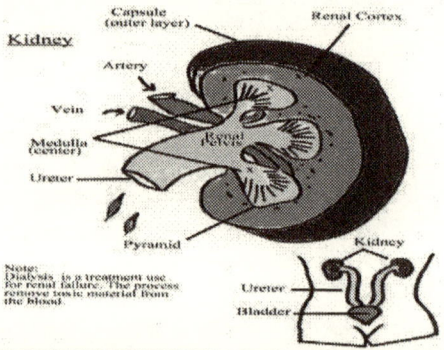

Most common kidney disorders:

Calculus- *there are varies types of stone formation, however these hard like rocks are mostly composed of mineral salt and other chemical present in the urine. Stones can be found in the bladder, gallbladder, ureters and kidney. Stones lead to obstructions, which can damage organs and caused infections. Most common factors are: Dehydration, high Intake of calcium, and metabolic disorders.*

Page 32

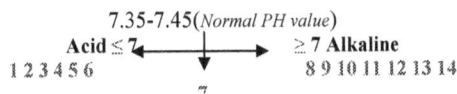

7.35-7.45(*Normal PH value*)

Acid ≤ 7 ⟵ ⟶ ≥ 7 Alkaline

1 2 3 4 5 6   8 9 10 11 12 13 14

7

Abnormal Urine

Protein (*Proteinuria*)	1st Signs Renal Disease
Glucose (*Glucosuria)*	Signs of diabetes
Ketone	Diets, diabetes
Bilirubin/(*Bilirubinuria*)	Liver disease
Blood (*Hematuria*)	Kidney disease, trauma
Urobilinogen	Liver disease
WBC *(Pyuria)*	UTI- infection

Note: Normal daily urine output ranges from 1,000-1500 cc or (*1-1½- Quart*) depending on fluid intake. Urine is composed of **95%** water and **5%** dissolved Chemicals Such as: Urea, uric acid, creatinine, ammonia, sodium chloride, calcium, Urochrome, sulfates, Phosphate, and Hydrogen ions.

Urination	Possible causes:
Polyuria(*Excessive)*	Diabetes, Kidney disease, diuretic such as: Caffeine, or digitalis.
Oliguria(*Little urine)*	Dehydration caused by Fever, diarrhea, vomiting, or heart disease
Anuria *(none)*	Acute nephritis (*kidney infections*), Uremia,
Nocturia	Urination during the night usually cause by too much fluid intake.
Dysuria	Painful or difficult urination, most common cause is UTI infections.

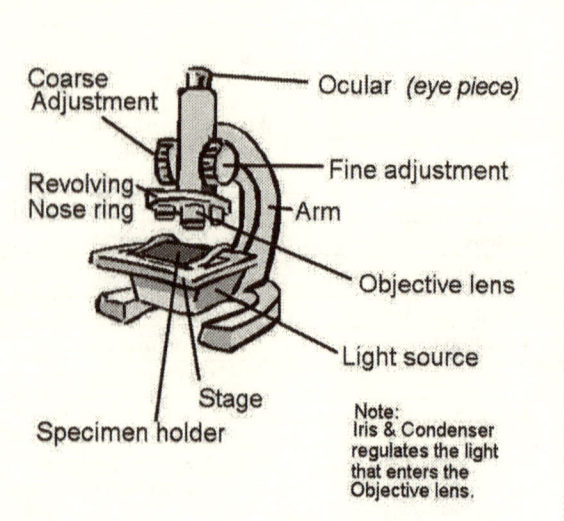

Coarse Adjustment

Ocular *(eye piece)*

Fine adjustment

Revolving Nose ring

Arm

Objective lens

Light source

Stage

Specimen holder

Note:
Iris & Condenser regulates the light that enters the Objective lens.

<u>Microscope-</u> it's an optical instrument use to view small objects closer with the used of magnifying lenses. It's used in laboratory to identifying pathogenic microorganism, counting blood cells, platelets, urinary cast and crystals and other body fluids. There many types of microscope from simple to High powered Electron microscope. Microscopes are either monocular *(One eye piece)* or binocular *(Two eye piece)*. The Objective lens magnify objects, the Smallest lens had a power of 10x, the medium lens has power of 40x and the largest is call the submersion lens because it can be submerge in oil, it has the power to magnify 100x. There are many different styles and shape of Microscope however the component is basically the same.

Types of equipment and functions

Autoclave – machine used for sterilization of medical instruments, by using pressurized stream or gas.

Ultrasonic cleaners- clean and disinfect instruments by using chemicals and sounds waves.

Glucometer-device used to measure blood sugar levels, most often used by the Diabetic patient to monitor daily sugar.

AED (*automatic external defibrillation*) - machine used in emergency cases of fibrillation rhythm, it gives electrical shocks to the heart and reset it rhythm.

Audio meter- Machine used for testing hearing.

Otoscope- A device used for looking into the human ear.

Snelle charts- used to test the vision for distance performance.

Ishahara book- used to test for color vision and color blindness.

Opthalmoscope- instrument for looking into dilate eye to see the retina located in the back of the eye and blood vessels.

Tonometer- it measures the pressure in the eye, used in Glaucoma testing.

Droppler- instrument used to magnify pulses and fetal heart sounds.

Spirometer- a device used to measure lung capacity; test is helpful to detect early lung diseases, it's recommended for smoker and COPD patients.

Holter Monitor- Portable Electrocardiography device used to monitor and record 24 hour cardiac activity.

Centrifuge- A common laboratory machine that uses spinning motion to separate blood cell from plasma and other body fluids.

CT scan-CAT- CT-(*Computerized Tomography)* or **CAT-**(*computerized axial tomography)* combines the used of computer and X ray pictures.

MRI- Magnetic resonance imaging- is a scanner that provides high quality cross sectional images of the organs without x-rays or radiation. It uses Magnetic and radio waves to get a picture .*Caution:* the used of electrical devices white testing is dangerous for example Pacemaker.

Nebulizer- A machine that delivers fast drugs in an aerosol form, often used during an asthma attack to administered Bronchodilator into the lungs.

Pacemaker- it can be external or implanted it's a device that supplies electrical impulse to the heart to maintain the regular beat.

Mammography- low dose of X-rays pictures used to detect breast cancer.

Laparoscope- a type of endoscope used to view the abdominal cavity.

Endoscope- A tube like instrument with lens and light used to view organs and body cavities.

Sigmoidoscope- a type of endoscope inserted via rectum, used to view the sigmoid colon.

Types of Procedures

Angioplasty- procedure used to open block or narrow blood vessels, this process introduces a balloon catheter into the affected area, then it inflated a few time to stretch and widen, process done under anesthetic.

Biopsy- is the removal of a sample tissue or cells for studies purpose.

Colostomy- An artificial Opening created from the large intestine to the surface of the skin for waste collection e.g. (*bowel*).

Hemodialysis- A machine that act as an artificial kidney, used to filter and remove waste product from the blood of patients with renal failure

Hysterectomy- Surgical removal of the UTERUS. Female sterilization.

Vasectomy- Male sterilization- process severs the pathway of sperm cells (*vas deferens)* preventing escape and union with female egg.

Papanicolaou test- Pap smear test, the scraping of the cervix for cell analyzing. *E.g. level of Hormones, Herpes or cancer.*

Amniocentesis- process done under local anesthesia, it's an invasive procedure which consist of a hollow needle penetrating the Pregnant female amniotic sac and a sample of fluid is remove for laboratory testing, this procedure is used to detect abnormal fetus defect such as spinal bifida or genetics disorders such as Down's *syndrome*, it can also identified unborn genders.

Tonsillectomy- The surgical removal of tonsils a pair of oval mass in the back of throat, made of lymphoid tissue and part of the *Lymphatic system*.

Spinal tap or Lumbar puncture- is an invasive procedure where a hollow needle is used to extract Cerebrospinal fluid, to test for disease such as meningitis, or to inject medications.

Endotracheal intubations- Is a tube inserted into the trachea to maintain open airway and deliver oxygen into the lungs of a comatose, anesthetize or patient with respiratory compromise.

Appendectomy- surgically removal of the appendix due to an acute appendicitis (*inflammation of appendix*), this emergencies often cause by an obstruction of feces or *Pinworm infestation*. Immediate surgery is required to prevent rupture and contamination of the abdominal cavity causing *Peritonitis*.

Tracheostomy-(*stoma)* an opening through neck into trachea (*windpipe*).

NG-Nasogastric Tube –feeding tube via the nostrils into the stomach.

Splenectomy- The surgical removal of the spleen.

Parts of a syringe

Route	Gauge	Length
Intradermal	27- 28	⅜ inches
Subcutaneous	25-26	½ , ⅝ inches
Intramuscular	20- 23	1 –3 inches

The width of a needle is called gauge.
Needles ranges in size from 14 the
largest to 28 the Smallest.

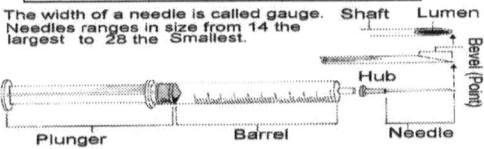

Type of injection:	Sites:
Intramuscular injection is inserted at a 90°angle into the muscle. *Example:* Penicillin	Deltoid, Gluteus medius (*buttock*), Vastus lateralis-*(Upper outer thigh)*
Subcutaneous injection, it injected at a 45°angle. *Example:* Vaccines, Insulin.	Abdomen, anterior thigh, upper outer arm & Subscapular portion of back.
Intradermal is administered just under the skin The Epidermis.	Upper chest, upper back & Foreman *Example: (tuberculin)*

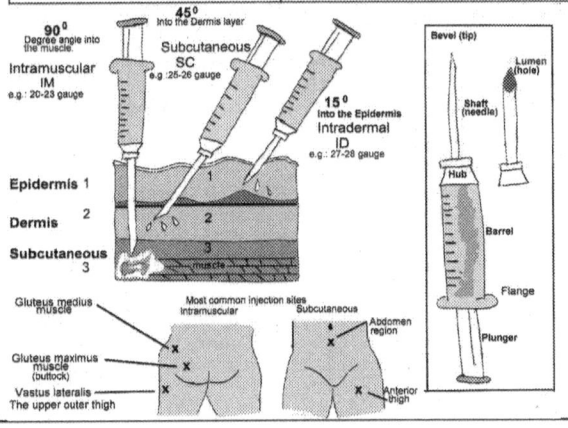

Immunization

Immunization is a form of protecting the body from certain diseases or infections. Vaccination is to administer a small weak dose or of a specified disease to stimulate the body to create antibodies, which will be store and will fight later when exposed to the disease. *Note:* Vaccination is composed of dead or weak microorganism and will not cause the disease.

DPT Viral & Bacterial *(Airborne)*	2, 4, 6, Months and a booster at age 5 years
MMR/ viral *(Body fluids, Airborne, object)*	12, 15 months, 4- 6 years
Influenza/ viral Airborne *(Droplet)*	2, 4, 6 months
Hepatitis B/ viral *(Contact, Fluids)*	Birth to 2 # 1 2 to 4 months # 2 6 months # 3
Varicella/ viral *(Airborne, direct contact)*	12, 18 months
Pneumococcal *(Droplet)*	2, 4, 6 months
Polio/ viral *(Airborne/ fluids)*	2, 4, months Booster 4 - 6 years

- **Rubella:** -*(German measles)* incubation time is 14-21 days, symptoms may resemble a flu with red rash over body, fever & swollen lymph nodes , possible complication include ear infections, and pneumonia.
- **Measles** *(Rubeolla)* incubation 10-12 days acquire by direct contact & body fluids.
- **Pertussis:** *(whooping cough)* respiratory infections transmitted airborne and contact, incubation period is 5-21 days.
- **Chicken Pox:** - *(Varicella)* 10-14 days incubation period, itching skin rash, red blister and scab.
- **Polio-** a viral infection of the intestines that affect the central nervous system which can lead to paralysis.
- **Mumps:** - has an incubation period of 14-21 days, possible complications are Meningitis and Encephalitis. Mumps is an Inflammation of the parotid and salivary Glands. S/S: includes swollen painful gland under jaw & cheek, fever, headache, and difficulty breathing.
- **Tetanus-** is a bacterium found in soil, it's enter a puncture wound *e.g.* gunshot or stabbing, the toxin causes muscle stiffness such as *Lockjaw*.
- **Hepatitis-** Caused by a virus that can damage the liver, other organ or even caused of death, transmitted by contact, blood, & body fluids.

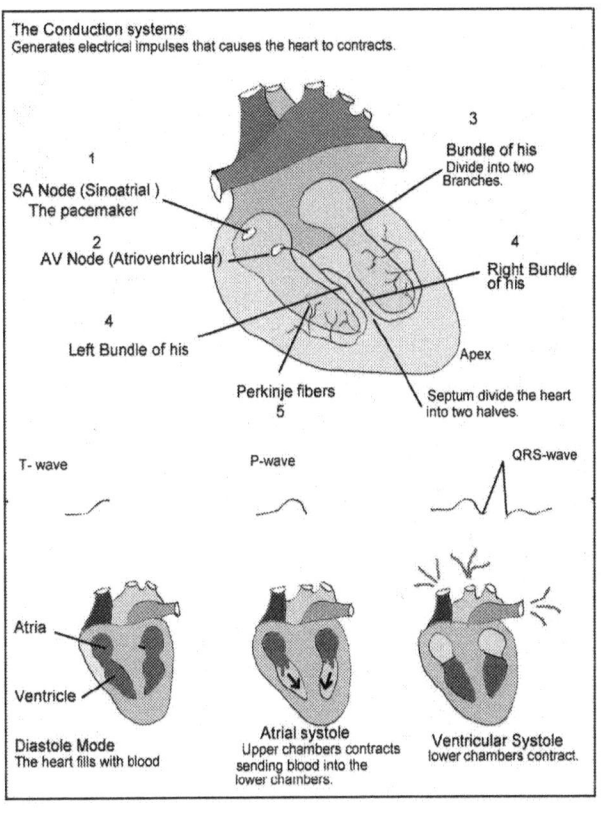

The Conduction systems
Generates electrical impulses that causes the heart to contracts.

1
SA Node (Sinoatrial)
The pacemaker

2
AV Node (Atrioventricular)

3
Bundle of his
Divide into two
Branches.

4
Right Bundle
of his

4
Left Bundle of his

Apex

Perkinje fibers
5

Septum divide the heart
into two halves.

T- wave

P-wave

QRS-wave

Atria

Ventricle

Diastole Mode
The heart fills with blood

Atrial systole
Upper chambers contracts
sending blood into the
lower chambers.

Ventricular Systole
lower chambers contract.

EKG & Lead Placement
EKG / ECG

Lead	Site	Colors
V1	Fourth Intercostals Space on the right side of body	Red
V2	Fourth intercostals on the left side of body	Yellow
V3	Midway between V2 & V4 on the left side	Green
V4	Fifth intercostals space left midclavicular line	Blue
V5	Fifth intercostals left anterior axillary (*Armpits*)	Orange
V6	Fifth intercostals left midaxillary line.	Purple

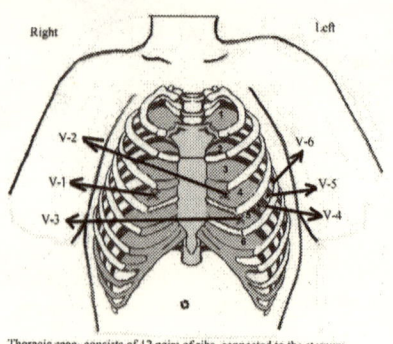

Thoracic cage- consists of 12 pairs of ribs, connected to the sternum by means of costal cartilage (exception for the floating ribs). Thoracic cage protect the heart, lungs and blood vessels.

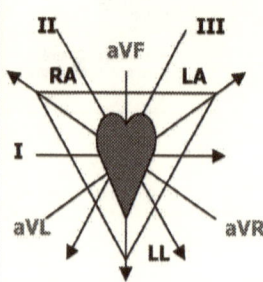

The Einthoven Triangle
Reference point for 12 lead ECG, using 3 limbs electrodes.

Most common EKG rhythms

Sinus Tachycardia

This condition is when the heart rates are abnormally fast over 100 beats per minutes. Most common causes: caffeine, exercise, heart disease, fever and drugs.

Most common Symptoms:

- Palpitations
- Breathless and lightheadedness.

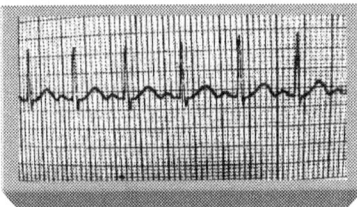

Sinus Bradycardia

Bradycardia rhythm –it occurs when the heart rate is slower than normal, less than 60 beats per minutes. Is most common type of arrhythmia seen in patients who have suffered a heart attack, athletes and in people who suffers from Hypothyroidism.

Most common Symptoms:

- Fatigue, Weakness, and fainting

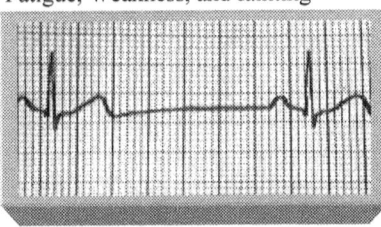

Atrial Fibrillation

A-FIB is an Irregular heart beat; which causes the **upper** heart chambers (*Atrium*) to beat fast and irregular *e.g.* (*300 to 500*) beats per minutes. Most common arrhythmia found in the elderly and people with Hyperthyroidism. This Rhythm is considered a shockable emergency.

Signs & symptoms:

- Rapid & irregular pulse

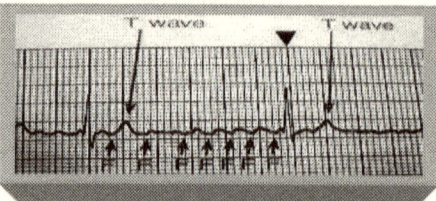

Ventricular Fibrillation

V-FIB occurs when the electrical impulse in the heart becomes chaotic and disorganized, causing the contractions of the **lower** chambers to beat rapid and irregular. The heart begins to quivers like a bag of worms. This emergency can be corrected with early defibrillation.

Signs & Symptoms:

- Absent pulse, blood pressure, Loss of consciousness
- Dilated pupils, cyanosis and seizures.

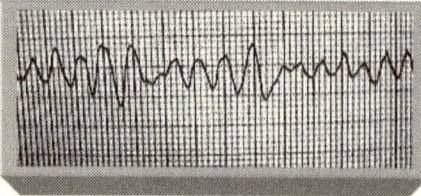

EKG/ ECG
Horizontally each box represents 0.4 seconds (*Time*).

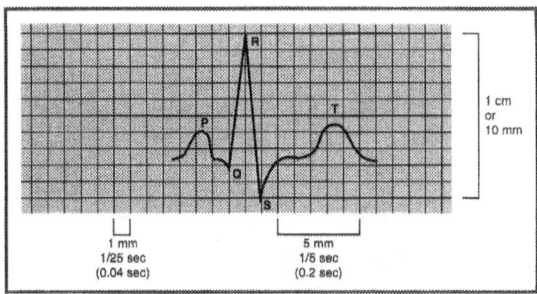

Cardiac cycle- The term refers to one complete heart beat, which consist of depolarization *(contraction)*, repolarization (*recovery*) and polarization (*Relaxation*) of the heart.
Understanding the WAVES
P *wave* –first small wave seen, rounded, upright (*positive)*
        represents Atrial depolarized followed by contractions.
Q- *wave-* Follows **P** always negative pointing below baseline.
        wave is small and the first wave of the complex.
R- *wave-* Follows **Q,** always positive, pointing upward above
        baseline.
S- *wave-* Follows **R** always negative.
QRS-*wave-* combine all three deflections which represent ventricular
        depolarization.
T *-wave* – rounded, represent ventricular repolarization

Note: there is no Atrial repolarization because is too small of wave and it shadow by the large QRS wave.
* Normal duration of a complex is less than .12 seconds.
INTREPRETING EKG/ ECG
- Six second method: In six second count the number of Complexes QRS x 10.
- Small boxes: count the number of small boxes between R –R then Multiply by 1500
- Large boxes: count the number of large boxes between R-R Then divide into 300.

Other: EKG Rhythms

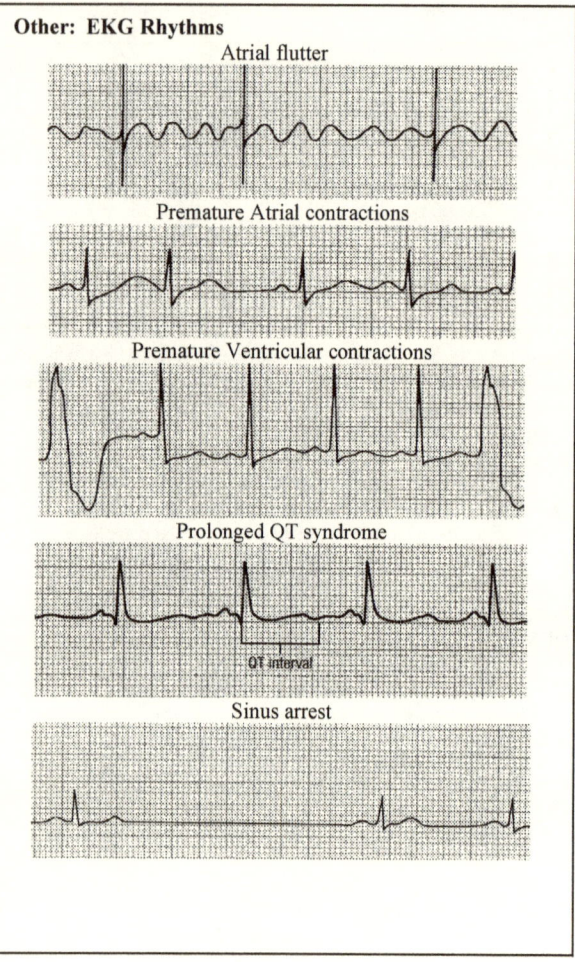

Atrial flutter

Premature Atrial contractions

Premature Ventricular contractions

Prolonged QT syndrome

QT interval

Sinus arrest

Digestive systems

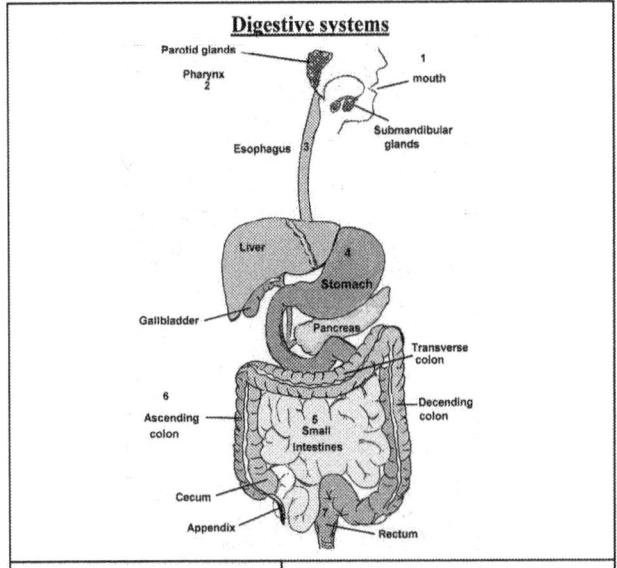

Parotid glands
Pharynx 2
Esophagus 3
Liver
Stomach 4
Gallbladder
Pancreas
Ascending colon 6
Cecum
Appendix
mouth 1
Submandibular glands
Transverse colon
Decending colon
Small Intestines 5
Rectum

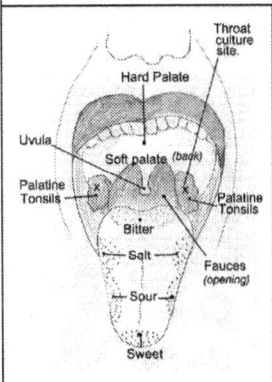

Throat culture site.
Hard Palate
Uvula
Soft palate *(back)*
Palatine Tonsils
Palatine Tonsils
Bitter
Salt
Sour
Sweet
Fauces *(opening)*

Digestion is the process of breaking down food, for cell absorption, it begin in the (1) mouth where the teeth crushed food and salivary gland secrets saliva, then the tongue pushed food into the (2) Pharynx leading into the (3) esophagus a long tube like pathway connected into the (4) stomach, In the stomach food is mix with gastric juices, after 3-4 hour The food enters the (5) Small intestine, the principal center for absorption. The small intestine is divide into three the Duodenum, Jejunum and ileum, finally it moves into the(6) large intestine where liquids are absorbed final ,and waste is sent to the(7) rectum then it exit through (8)Anus.

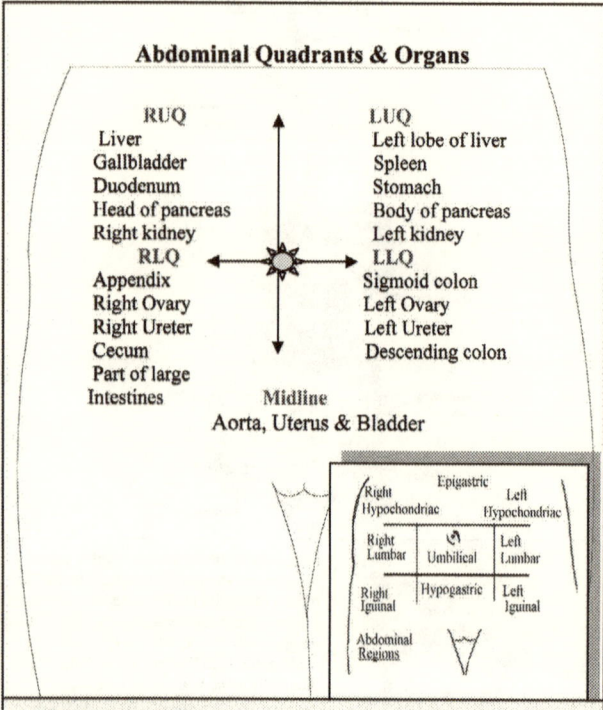

Abdominal Quadrants & Organs

RUQ
Liver
Gallbladder
Duodenum
Head of pancreas
Right kidney

RLQ
Appendix
Right Ovary
Right Ureter
Cecum
Part of large
Intestines

LUQ
Left lobe of liver
Spleen
Stomach
Body of pancreas
Left kidney

LLQ
Sigmoid colon
Left Ovary
Left Ureter
Descending colon

Midline
Aorta, Uterus & Bladder

Right Hypochondriac	Epigastric	Left Hypochondriac
Right Lumbar	Umbilical	Left Lumbar
Right Iguinal	Hypogastric	Left Iguinal

Abdominal Regions

Abdominal Organs:

Hollow organs- *are tubes or sacs containing fluids that when injured leaks, causing contamination and infections. E.g. Stomach, gallbladder, duodenum, Large intestines, small intestines, & Bladder.*
Solids organs- *are made of a firm mass of tissue, when injured they tend to bleed profusely. E.g. Diaphragm, Spleen, Liver, Pancreas & Kidney.*

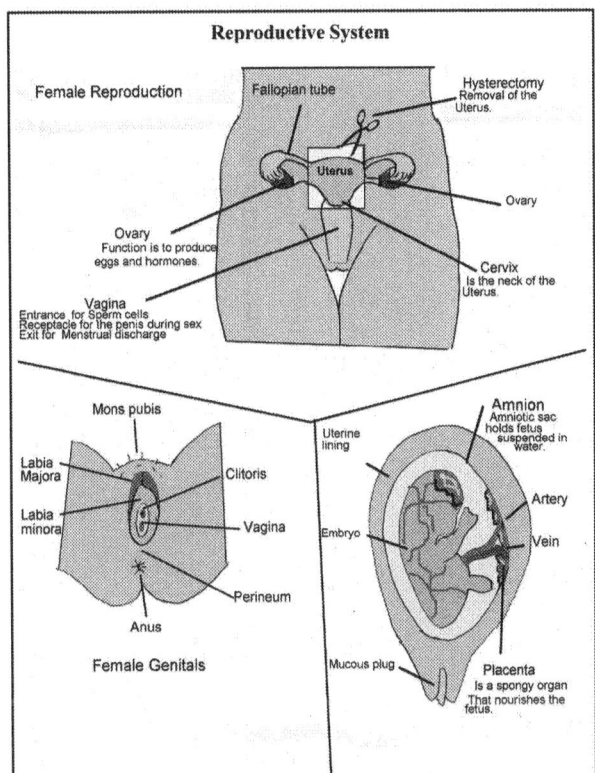

Reproductive System

Female Reproduction

Fallopian tube

Hysterectomy
Removal of the Uterus.

Uterus

Ovary

Ovary
Function is to produce eggs and hormones.

Cervix
Is the neck of the Uterus.

Vagina
Entrance for Sperm cells
Receptacle for the penis during sex
Exit for Menstrual discharge

Mons pubis

Labia Majora

Clitoris

Labia minora

Vagina

Perineum

Anus

Female Genitals

Uterine lining

Amnion
Amniotic sac holds fetus suspended in water.

Artery

Embryo

Vein

Mucous plug

Placenta
Is a spongy organ That nourishes the fetus.

The Female Reproductive & other

The purpose of the reproductive systems is to produce offspring. The female produces eggs *(ova)* and the hormones estrogen and progesterone in her ovaries. The union of an egg and sperm produces a single cell, which through growth and division the new individual developed. Menstruation is the shedding of the lining of the uterus (*The Endometrium*), caused by low level of hormones and no fertilization of an egg. The process causes bleeding and cramping, the length of flow varies on individual, usually 3-7 days. The lining rebuilt itself and the cycle repeats every 28 days. Menstruation begins at puberty and end with menopause. Menopause is due to lack of or changing in hormones levels cause by disease or the aging process.

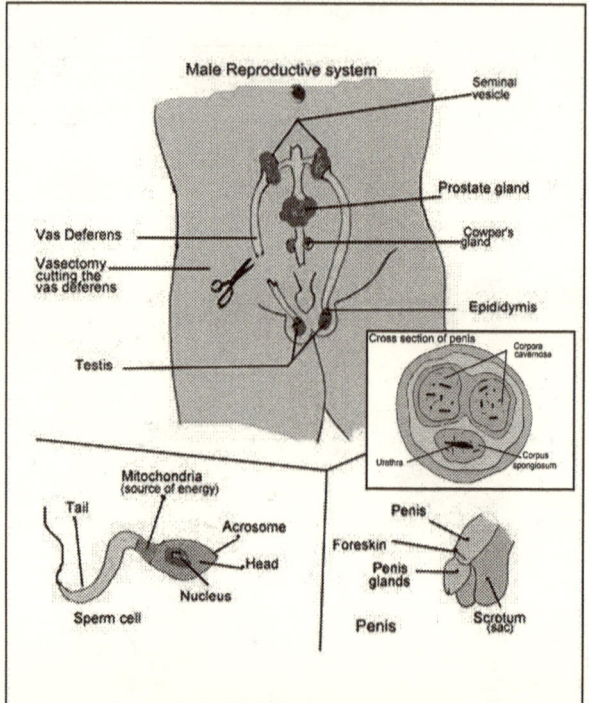

The male Reproductive System

The male organs are found in and out of the body. Inside are glands such as the Prostate and tubes like structures, which are the pathway of sperm cells, called the Vas deferens. Outside is the Penis and behind it there a bag of skin that hangs call the scrotum, inside suspended are the testes two glands responsible for the production of sperms cells. *Note:* Sperms cells can live in the female fallopian tubes for up to 48 hour in which it can still fertilized an egg. Vasectomy is the cutting and blockage of the sperm pathway the Vas deferens.

Alcohol and the Body

Alcohol is a drug and even in small amount it affects the body and mental function. It can cause damage to organs such as e.g. *Liver* and *heart* or it can lead to early death.

Long-term effect of alcohol on the body

Liver	Urinary system
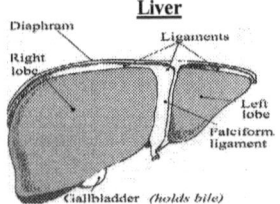	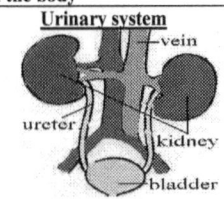
Causes: The Liver is the main organ that metabolized alcohol from the blood , long term drinking leads to Hepatitis, cirrhosis and Liver cancer	*Causes*: Alcohol increase urine output causing dehydration, long term abuse lead to Renal failure.

Brain Function	Digestive system
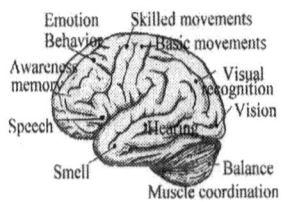	*Causes*: Gastritis and ulcers Note: *Ulcers*-are open sore, It may be shallow or deep crater like, usually inflamed and painful.
	Reproductive
	Causes: Small amount Increases sexual behavior, long term use leads to Impotence.
	Skin
Causes: depresses the Nervous system, prolonged usage causes permanently impairs brain and nerves.	*Causes*: Facial flushing.

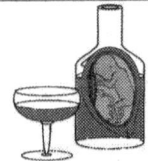

Note:

Alcohol can cause damage to the fetus, this condition is known as Fetal Alcohol syndrome, the disorder consist of facial abnormalities Such as cleft lip and palate, small eyes and jaw, heart defect, abnormal development, and low birth weight.

Caffeine *(Stimulant)*

Caffeine is a stimulant. Within few minutes of consumption it produces a hype reaction in the body and Organs. It causes sweating, tremors, and talkativeness. Caffeine is often used as a diet ingredient because it can suppress appetite.

Effects on the body

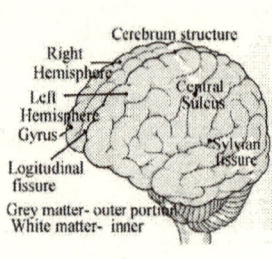	In small quantity it stimulates the brain, reduce drowsiness and fatigue. In large amount- causes over stimulation, anxiety, irritability, restlessness and insomnia.
	In small amount increased blood pressure and heart rate. Large amount- causes palpitations.
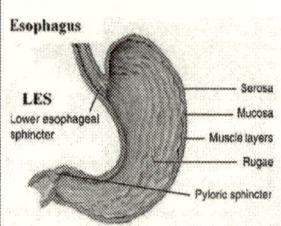	Small amount -can help digestion by increasing stomach acid. Large amount it causes abdominal pain and nausea. Prolonged used and abuse can lead to ulcers.
	In the kidney it acts as a diuretic, causing increase urination.

Cocaine/Hydrochloride

Cocaine a crystalline drug derived from the coca leaves used as a central nervous system stimulant. It causes excitement, restlessness, hallucination, increased pulse respiration and heart rate. Cocaine was once used as a tropical anesthetic applied to the mucous membrane for minor surgeries, however because of its potential for abuse it was replaced by other local anesthetic. Regular inhaling can damage the lining of the nose causing ulcers, bleeding, and also becoming sensitive; continue use can lead to psychological dependency and psychosis. Overdose can cause seizures, and cardiac arrest. "Crack" it a purified form of cocaine, it produces a more rapid and intense reaction, which wears off quickly. It has caused deaths due to it adverse effects on the heart.

Common used Drug:	
Categories:	**Example:**
Two type of stimulants: Nerve Stimulant: Reduce drowsiness, & increase alertness. Respiratory Stimulants: Act on the respiratory center in the brain stem	Amphetamines, and Caffeine.
Depressants:	Alcohol, & Barbiturates
Psychedelics:	LSD (*Produce Hallucination*)
Narcotics (*Analgesics*): Type of painkillers	Cocaine, Heroin, codeine, and morphine

The DEA *(Drug enforcement Agency)* has developed a method to regulate & controlled drugs under a 5 schedule Program.

I Schedule *Drugs with no medical purpose*	Illegal, high potential for abused e.g. Heroin, LSD, Marijuana, mescaline & peyote or drugs classified as Orphan drugs.
II Schedule *Drugs with medical purpose, and high abuse potential.*	Various Narcotics e.g.: Opium, morphine, methadone, Stimulants e.g. Cocaine, amphetamines, Depressants e.g. barbiturates.
III Schedule *Drugs with medical purpose, less potential for abuse.*	Aspirin & Tylenol with codeine, amphetamines like substance.
IV Schedule	Minor Tranquilizers and Hypnotics Drugs, Equanil, Valium, Librium, Dalmane, Darvon.
V Schedule	Miscellaneous drugs/ over the counter

51

Respiration -is the process of inhaling oxygen and exhaling waste product such as carbon dioxide. Oxygen is a clear odorless gas that is essentials for life. Cells obtain their energy mainly from metabolized glucose and oxygen. The organs responsible for breathing are the lungs two spongy like mass located in the thoracic cavity, encased in a sac called the pleura. Respirations begins when oxygen enters the mouth and nose, then it moves into the 1-Pharynx, enter the epiglottis which is the trap door that prevent food from entering the lungs. And then the 2-Larynx which contains the vocal cords ,and then 3- the trachea also call the *windpipe*, down into the lungs and then the 4-Bronchus tubes which divide into two branches, left and right and then it enters the 5- Bronchioles, and finally the 6- alveoli where gasses are exchanged in the capillaries

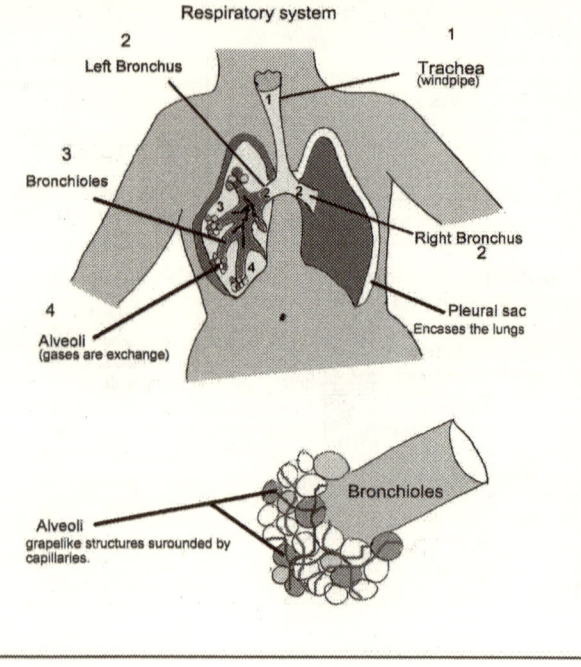

Respiratory system

2
Left Bronchus

1
Trachea
(windpipe)

3
Bronchioles

Right Bronchus
2

4
Alveoli
(gases are exchange)

Pleural sac
Encases the lungs

Bronchioles

Alveoli
grapelike structures surounded by capillaries.

<u>Asthma</u>

It's a chronic respiratory disorder that causes, bronchospasm, narrowing of the bronchial tubes, and difficulty breathing. It's an allergic reaction to something inhaled, ingested or injected, it can also be triggered by infections, Emotional factors, such as stress or anxiety, seasonal, weather such as (*cold*) or exercise. Asthma also has a strong hereditary factor. An attack can be sudden or mild, most common treatments are Bronchodilators and removal of allergens, in severe emergency an epinephrine injection, and steroid is administered , hospitalization may be require.

<u>Most common Signs & Symptoms</u>:

- Rapid pulse (*Tachycardia*)
- DOB/ Difficult Breathing, wheezing
- Coughing
- Diaphoresis (*sweating*)
- Cyanosis (*bluish skin color due to lack of oxygen*)
- Tightness in the chest
- Unable to speak

<u>*Note:*</u>
Most common Allergens responsible for asthma are: pollens, house dust, mold, roaches, animal fur, dander, feathers, respiratory infections such as: Bronchitis, The flu, strong odors such as perfumes, tobacco smoke or others air pollutant, food e.g. peanuts, shellfish or drugs such as Aspirin and x-ray dyes.

Chronic Obstructive pulmonary diseases
(Lung disease)

COPD- is a combination of chronic lung disease Such as: Asthma, Bronchitis and Emphysema. It's a condition that persistently disrupts the airflow of oxygen. Causes can be damage to the Alveoli ,microscopic air sacs in the lungs where gas are exchange in the capillaries surrounding it, or changes to the Bronchi tubes & Bronchioles. Patient with COPD are unable to exchanged gases and eliminated waste such as Carbon dioxide, they are hunched forward, often hyperventilate, and their chest appear to be shaped like a barrel.

Most common sign & symptoms:
* Difficulty Breathing and wheezing.

Bronchitis- Is an Inflammation of the bronchi caused by a bacterium. Repeated infections cause the wall of the Bronchi and Bronchioles to change, thicken and narrow with mucus. Condition most commons in smokers.

Emphysema- is a condition affecting the Alveoli. The sac become distended and may burst with trapped air, some merge reducing oxygen, most common among smokers.

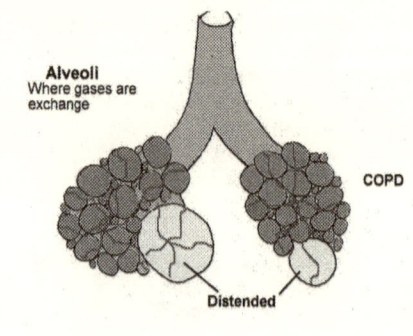

Alveoli
Where gases are exchange

COPD

Distended

<u>Common Cold</u>

A cold is highly contagious, caused by a virus that causes
inflammation of the mucous membrane lining the nose &
throat.
Viruses are transmitted by hand-to-hand contact *(touch)*
and droplets expelled into the air by a sneezed or cough.
It can lead to secondary bacterial infections such as:
Bronchitis, sinusitis, otitis *(Ear infections)*, and
pneumonia. It can also aggravate existing respiratory
disorders such as asthma and Chronic Bronchitis.

Most common signs & Symptoms:

- Stuffy, runny nose
- Tickle or sore throat
- Headache, sneezing, watery eyes
- Cough, possible low-grade fever
- Possible Aching muscle & chills

Note:
*Cold without complication clear up within a week, most
recommended treatment is to increased fluids intake, bed
rest, an analgesic for pain, decongestant and frequent
hand wash. Seek medical advice before taking any
medication, or if symptoms get worst.*

Flu/ Influenza

It's a viral infection of the respiratory tracts,
(*The airway passage in the lungs*) Its spread by droplets
sneezed or coughs into the air, or by contact with
body fluid and contaminated objects. Flu can lead to
secondary bacterial infections Such as: Bronchitis,
Pneumonia, croup and other.
Flu can also aggravate other respiratory disorder
Such as: asthma. Usually flu clear within 7-10 days,
if no complication, most recommended treatment is
increased fluid intake , bed rest an analgesic for
pain and liquid diet.

Most Common Signs & Symptoms:

- Fever, Headaches
- Weakness, Chills, nausea
- Muscle aches, sneezing
- Loss of appetite, fatigue
- Cough, Possible diarrhea

Note:
*Flu shot: It won't prevent the flu, however It can reduced
complications especially for high-risk people with weak
immune system due to disease or a condition: for example:
Asthma, AIDS, diabetes, heart disease, lung disease and older
adult over 65.*

Headaches

Headaches are the most common type of pain. It may be acute or chronic; pain may be dull, throbbing or pressure. It can be cause by illness, infections such as: otitis, sinusitis, allergies, colds, fever, trauma, visions problems or it can be hereditary as in *Migraines*. Headache can also be trigger by, diets, poor posture, certain food like chocolate or additives, noise and hangovers. Headaches are the results of vessels contraction and changes in the brain chemical. Most common types of headache:

Migraines- a migraine begins when nerve cells send out impulses to the blood vessels, causing constriction, followed by dilatation of these vessels and then the release of inflammatory substances that causes the pain.

Most common signs & Symptoms:
- Light, noise sensitivity, nausea, vomiting
- Loss of appetite, abdominal upset
- Blur vision and irritability

Sinus Headache- is an inflammation of the nasal cavities, which causes pressure and severe pain behind the cheekbones, forehead and bridge of the nose. Pain intensifies with certain head movement. *Symptoms may include*: fever & facial swelling most common cause is allergies.

Tension Headache- Is the most common type of headache, often caused by tightening of the muscle in the head neck, and shoulders. Most common triggers are stress and poor postures.

Hormones Headache- is caused by changing Hormones levels during menstruation, menopause, and pregnancy.

CVA / Stroke

CVA <u>Cerebral Vascular accident</u> is cause by a disruption of blood supply to the brain causing tissue death, due to hemorrhage, a blockage caused by a thrombus which is fat or blood clot or an embolism which is a piece of traveling clot or an air bubble. Stroke may lead to complications such as: Paralysis, affect speech, thought processes, behavior and other brain function.

<u>Most common Signs & Symptoms:</u>

- LOC/ loss of consciousness, rapid pulse
- Unequal Pupils, Possible seizures
- Difficulty breathing, (*snoring*)
- Numbness, Weakness, paralysis one side
- Sudden Headache, nausea or vomiting
- Blur vision, Dizziness, confusion
- Loss of bladder and bowel control
- Difficulty swallowing & speech
- Elevated Blood pressure

<u>**Factors that increase the risk of a stroke includes**</u>: Age, high blood pressure, ateriosclerosis disease, heart disease, diabetes, smoking, polycythemia (*high levels of RBC*), Hyperlipidemia (*High level of fat in blood*) and the used of estrogens found in birth control pills. <u>**TIA's**</u> *Transient Ischemic attacks* also called mini strokes, is a condition often confused as a stroke because symptoms are alike however unlike the stroke, TIA causes no permanent damage and full recovery is expected. TIA's are, warning that the brain is being deprived of oxygen and blood; with early diagnosis and medical intervention it can prevent a more serious complication such as a stroke.

Meningitis

It's an Inflammation of the *Meninges*. It's diagnosed by an exam, spinal tap or lab test. It caused by Viruses, bacteria or parasites.
Viral meningitis- is mild with flu like symptoms. Recovery is expected within 1 to 2 weeks.
Bacterial meningitis -is severe; it will require intravenous antibiotic and hospitalization; it can lead to serious complications such as deafness, learning disabilities and death. Method of transmission: Airborne (*cough or sneeze*) and direct touch with body fluids or contaminated objects.
Most common signs & Symptoms:

- High Fever, severe headache
- Stiff neck, sensitivity to light
- Possible seizure, lethargy
- Nausea, Vomiting

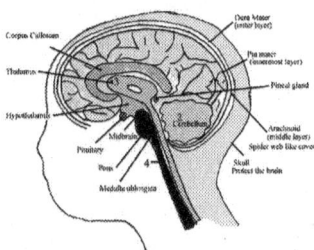

The Human Brain & spinal cord

The human brain weight about 3 pounds, is protected by three connecting membranes called meninges. The Dura mater is a tough and thick outer layer, the arachnoid is the middle layer which resemble a spider web covering the brain , and the Pia Mater which is the thinnest and contains blood vessels. The brain is divided into 4 -regions 1-Cerebrum The largest portion of the brain. 2-cerebellum (*2nd largest portion of the brain*), is responsible for maintaining balance, muscle coordination, and equilibrium3-Diencephalon (*regulate varies body functions*) and 4- the brain stem. The brain has two hemisphere divided by the deep Longitudinal fissure, both lobe communicated with each other by a band of white fibers call the Corpus Callosum.

Diabetes

Diabetes is a condition where the Pancreas is unable to produce sufficient or no Insulin. Insulin is a hormones needed to help cells absorbed sugar and use it for energy. Without Insulin sugar stays in the blood causing damage to organs and blood vessels. **Hyperglycemia** is the term refer to Its High level of glucose (*sugar*) greater than 200mg/dl in the blood, it can lead to Coma. Others causes are overeating, stress and infections.

Most Common Signs & Symptoms:
- Rapid pulse, normal or low BP
- Labored breathing, sighing
- Fruity breath odor (*Acetone*)
- Gradual Onset, Confusion
- Drowsiness, body aches, boils
- Extreme thirst (*Polydipsia*)
- Polyuria (*increased urination*)
- Blur vision, dry itching skin
- Stomach pain, nausea
- Vomiting
- Eventual Unconsciousness
- Tingling sensation, leg cramps
- Flushed skin

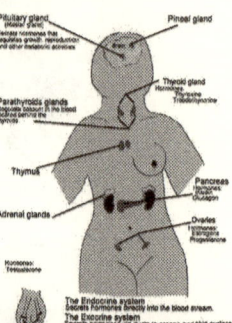

Diabetes complications: Hyperglycemia, Hypoglycemia, Heart and blood vessel diseases, retinopathy (eye damage or even blindness), Neuropathy (Nerve) Nephropathy (Kidney disease), and even amputation of limbs. Two type of Diabetes: Type I -insulin dependent and Type II- non-insulin, usually controlled by diets, and most common in obesity.

<u>Diabetes</u>

Hypoglycemia (*lead to Insulin Shock*)
Low level of glucose in the blood, Less than 60 mg/dl
it caused by too much Insulin in the body, too little
food, exercise or alcohol abuse.

<u>Most common Signs & Symptoms:</u>

- Sudden Onset, Anger
- Dizziness, and headache
- Normal BP, Full rapid pulse
- Fainting, seizures, palpitations
- Hunger, drooling, impaired vision
- Confusion, Disorientation, fatigue
- Staggering, poor coordination
- Nervous, diaphoresis (*sweating*)
- Cold, Pale, and clammy skin
- Eventual Unconsciousness

Recommended target range:

Before breakfast	80-120 mg/dl
No higher than 140	
Before bedtime	100-140 mg/dl
No higher than 160 mg/dl	
1-2 hour after meal goal is no higher than 180	

Merva Rivera

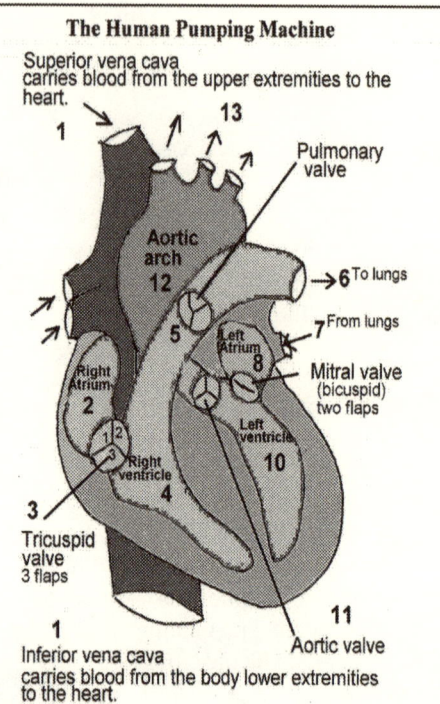

The Human Pumping Machine

Superior vena cava carries blood from the upper extremities to the heart.

1

13

Pulmonary valve

Aortic arch **12**

→**6** To lungs

5

7 From lungs

Left Atrium

Right Atrium **2**

8

Mitral valve (bicuspid) two flaps

Left ventricle

1 2
3

Right ventricle

4

10

3

Tricuspid valve 3 flaps

11

1

Inferior vena cava carries blood from the body lower extremities to the heart.

Aortic valve

The human heart- The heart is a muscular pump that provides the force needed to push blood throughout the body; it's about the size of a closed fist, weight about 9 ounces , it's a hollow muscular organ, situated in the thoracic cavity in the mediastinal region. The heart is encased in a sac called the Pericardium, it has three layers, the outer Epicardium made of a thin layer of connecting tissue, the myocardium middle layer made of Muscle tissue, and the Endocardium inner layer which is also the lining of the heart valve and blood vessels. The heart is dividing into two halves by the septum. It has 4 one way valves that keep blood flowing in one direction. The right side received deoxygenated blood from the body and the left oxygenate blood from the lungs.

MI-Myocardial Infarction
(Heart attack)

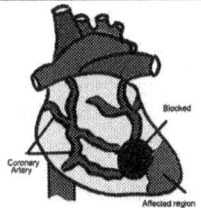

Sudden death of part of the heart muscle may be cause by a rupture vessels or blockage of a coronary artery that supplies blood & oxygen to the heart.

Most common Signs & Symptoms:

- Dyspnea (*difficult breathing*), Shallow
- Signs of shock, pale, cold clammy skin
- Diaphoresis (*profuse sweating*), Indigestion
- Tachycardia, low Blood pressure
- Crushing, squeezing pressure chest pain
- Nausea, Vomiting, weakness, anxiety
- Syncope, (*fainting*) Loss of consciousness
- Pain not relieved by rest or nitroglycerin
- Pain radiate to neck, jaw or arm
- Extreme apprehension

Nitroglycerin: Is a vasodilator, administered under the tongue (*sublingual*), it dilates arteries which increase blood flow and oxygen to the heart. Primary used for Angina & CHF. Most common Side effects include Falling BP, Syncope & Nausea. *Precaution:* Never administer if BP is less than 120 systolic.

Risk Factors: *Family history of heart disease, Smokers, stress High Blood pressure, age, Diabetes, high cholesterol, obesity and physical inactivity.*

Distinguishing
Angina from Myocardial Infarction

Angina Pectoris	Vs.	Myocardial Infarctions
Substernal / across chest	Pain Location	Same
Neck, jaw or arms	Pain radiates To	Same
A pressures or squeezing sensation	Pain	Same but more intense
Usually last 8-10 minutes	Duration	Last longer than 30 minutes
None	Other Symptoms	Sweating, weakness, nausea and pale skin color
Extreme weather, exertion, stress and heavy meals	Precipitating Factors	Often None
Stop physical activity, reduced stress and exertion or nitroglycerin	Relief	None seek medical emergencies for Evaluation

Note:
All chest pain should be evaluation at once, treated as a heart attack and emergencies procedures should be taken.

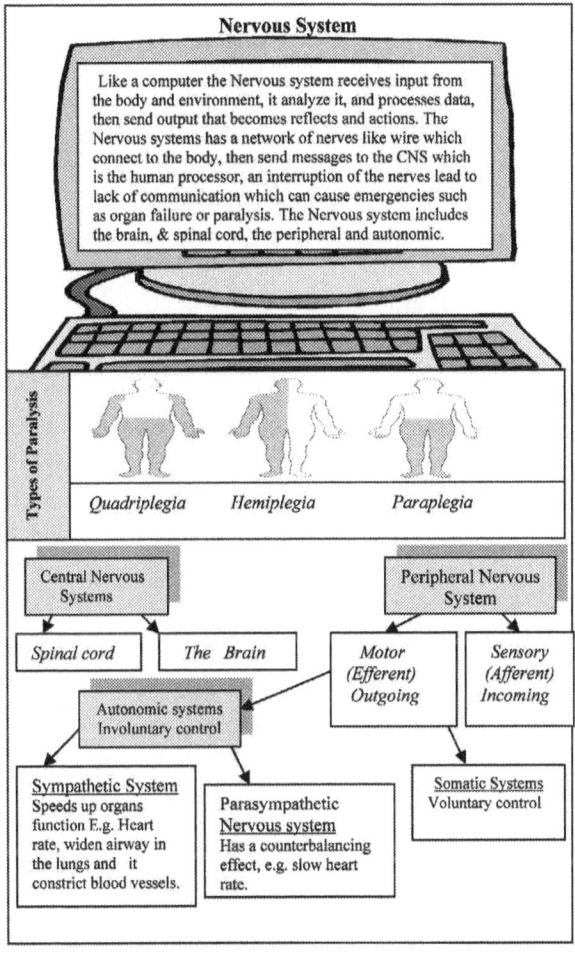

Nervous System

Like a computer the Nervous system receives input from the body and environment, it analyze it, and processes data, then send output that becomes reflects and actions. The Nervous systems has a network of nerves like wire which connect to the body, then send messages to the CNS which is the human processor, an interruption of the nerves lead to lack of communication which can cause emergencies such as organ failure or paralysis. The Nervous system includes the brain, & spinal cord, the peripheral and autonomic.

Types of Paralysis

Quadriplegia   *Hemiplegia*   *Paraplegia*

Central Nervous Systems

Peripheral Nervous System

Spinal cord   *The Brain*

Motor (Efferent) Outgoing   *Sensory (Afferent) Incoming*

Autonomic systems Involuntary control

<u>Sympathetic System</u>
Speeds up organs function E.g. Heart rate, widen airway in the lungs and it constrict blood vessels.

Parasympathetic <u>Nervous system</u>
Has a counterbalancing effect, e.g. slow heart rate.

<u>Somatic Systems</u>
Voluntary control

Seizures/ Convulsions

It's a sudden episode of uncontrolled electrical disturbance in the brain. Seizures may be cause by many different neurological or medical problems, including, head trauma, Stroke, brain tumor, fever, toxic, diabetes, Infections such as Meningitis, alcohol withdrawal, drugs such as Cocaine & heroin, epilepsy, or lack of oxygen. There are two main types of seizures 1- *Petit mal-* (*absence seizures*) is a type of seizures that occurs with epilepsy it last only for a short period, and can happen several times during the day. The patient may appears to be daydreaming; sometimes attacks may even pass unnoticed without muscle movement.

2-*Grand mal-(Tonic clonic)* is a type of more serious seizures that can lead to unconsciousness patient may fall, have twitching of muscle and have no recollection on awakening.

Most common Signs & Symptoms:

- Convulsion, twitching of limbs
- LOC / Loss of consciousness, AMS
- Fever (*Febrile seizures*), blurred vision
- Headache, drowsiness, Confusion
- Foams at the mouth and drool
- Loss of bladder and bowel control
- Possible vomiting, clenching jaw

Warning! *During a seizure removed all harmful surrounding objects, never used restraint, and Do Not insert object into mouth, because it may break causing injuries of tooth and soft tissue, in addition it may cause obstructions. After an episode has ended place victim on his or her side and call 911 for Emergency treatment & evaluation. Monitor breathing because there is a high risk or arrest.*

Swallowed Poisons

Poison is any substance that causes harm to the body and organs function. Poison can be ingested (Swallowed), injected, absorbed or inhale.

Most common signs & Symptoms
- Difficulty breathing
- Sudden Abdominal Pain
- Cramping, Diarrhea
- Nausea or vomiting
- Burn, odor or stain around mouth if chemical
- Drowsiness or unconsciousness
- Near bye container
- Diaphoresis (*sweating*)

Check for ABC and monitor respiration

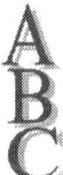

Airway- make sure is open, & no obstructions.

Breathing. -Check for chest to raise and fall and listen for respiration.

Circulation- check for a pulse.

Never- induce vomiting unless instructed by the Poison Control Center. If vomiting is recommended it should be done within 20 minutes of poisoning. Never give anything to drink, because some poison made activate faster with water, place victim on his or her left side to slow down absorption process. When transporting patient to hospital take empty container if available for fast identification and antidote.

Merva Rivera

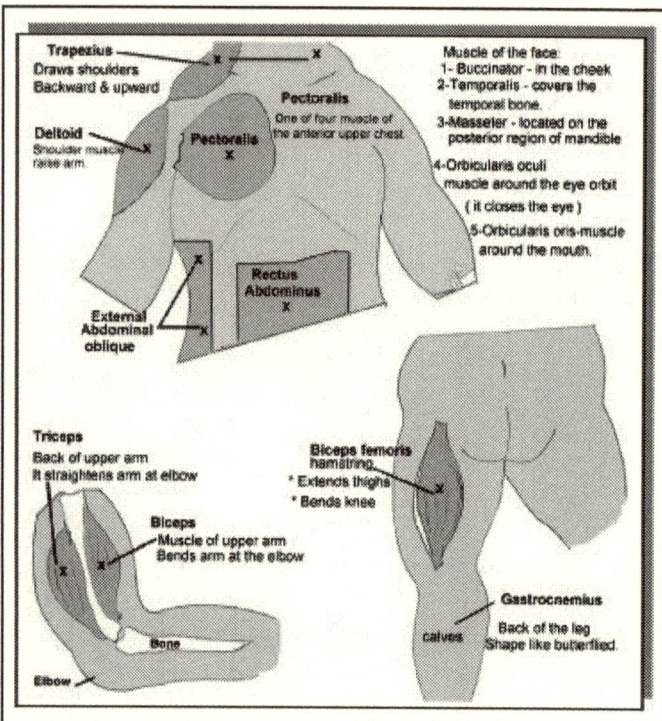

Trapezius —
Draws shoulders
Backward & upward

Deltoid -
Shoulder muscle
raise arm.

Pectoralis
One of four muscle of
the anterior upper chest

**External
Abdominal
oblique**

**Rectus
Abdominus**

Muscle of the face:
1- Buccinator - in the cheek
2-Temporalis - covers the
temporal bone.
3-Masseter - located on the
posterior region of mandible
4-Orbicularis oculi
muscle around the eye orbit
(it closes the eye)
5-Orbicularis oris-muscle
around the mouth.

Triceps
Back of upper arm
It straightens arm at elbow

Biceps
Muscle of upper arm
Bends arm at the elbow

Bone

Elbow

Biceps femoris
hamstring.
* Extends thighs
* Bends knee

Gastrocnemius
Back of the leg
Shape like butterfied.
calves

Muscle: The human body contains more than 600 muscles covering the
skeletal systems, It purpose is movement. There are three types of muscle.
1-Smooth or involuntary mostly make up the internal organs such as
stomach, intestines and blood vessels, we have no control.
2- Cardiac muscle found in the heart, and 3- Skeletal or striated muscle
which we can control movement.

Classifications of drugs & Example

Anti-inflammatory- use for treatments of arthritis and other inflammatory disorder example: Motrin, naproxen, and prednisone.

Antihistamine- Is a group of drugs used to block the histamine released by the body during an allergic reaction, symptoms includes: itching watery eyes, sneezing and Runny nose. *Example of the most common Antihistamine:*Benadryl, Allegra, Clarinex, Claridin-D, Nasonex, flonase.

Analgesics- are Drugs used to relieved pain, or fever, such as: aspirin, acetaminophen, Ibuprophen, or morphine.

Anticoagulants- (*Blood Thinner*) a group of drugs used to prevent coagulation of the blood. *Example:* Heparin, coumadin, warfarin sodium and aspirin

Antacids- A groups of drugs used to relieve the symptoms of Indigestion, Heartburn and inflammation cause by too much acid in the stomach. *Example:* Rolaids, Tums, Mylanta.

Antihypertensive- A group of drugs used to treat high blood pressure , it helps prevent complications such as Stroke, MI, and Kidney damage. *Example*: Enalapril, Atenolol, Verapramil, Adalat Procardia. Aldomet

Antibiotics- used to treat infections caused by bacteria.*Example*: Penicillin, Ceclor,tetracycline, amoxicillin, Augmentin.

Antiepileptic/ Anticonvulsants- Drug use for seizures for *example:* Dilantin, Phenobarbital, tegretol.

Antitussive-cough suppressants e.g. Robitussin

Bronchodilator- relaxes smooth muscle of bronchi and dilates the tubes, allowing more air to enter the lungs often used for asthma and other lungs disease. *Example*: ventolin, Abuterol, Proventil, Medrol,Intal, and theodur.

Cathartic (laxative*)* increases defecation (*bowel*)

Diuretic- Drugs that increased urination output decrease blood pressure, most often prescribes for certain heart conditions such as CHF and hypertension. *Example:* Lasix, furosemide, dyazide

Miotic-drugs causes pupil to contract.

Mydriatic- dilates pupils for examination.

Expectorant- increases secretions and mucus from the bronchial tubes, Primary use for upper respiratory tract congestion.

Merva Rivera

Anesthetic

Produce insensitivity to pain. Most common used Anesthetic.

Tropical anesthesia- applied on skin or mucous membrane e.g. *Abesol*

Local anesthetics-are injected into tissue or nerve. It produces a local effect of insensitivity.

General anesthetics- system action and produce sleep, It could be injected or inhale as in gas.

Drug	Common uses	Application	Action
Benzocaine	Skin irritation, toothache, teething pain and hemorrhoid	Cream, gel, spray, ointment	Rapid action short duration
Bupivacaine	As a nerve block _e.g._ Epidural	Injection	Medium action long duration
Cocaine	Minor surgery on the eyes, ear, nose and throat	Liquid or spray	Rapid action short duration
Lidocaine	Skin irritation, relieve pain during dental treatment, nerve block	Cream, ointment, spray or injection	Rapid action Medium Duration
Procaine	For relief of pain before surgery	Injections	Slow action slow duration
Tetracaine	Anal irritation, relive pain during dental treatment	Cream, ointment, spray, liquid, drops.	Rapid action medium to long duration

70

Glossary of Disease & conditions:

AIDS-Acquire immunodeficiency syndrome. One of the most deadly sexual diseases cause by a virus attack the immune system and weakens the capability to fight infections.

Anemia- Is the reduction of Red Blood cells, most common causes: Iron deficiency, Insufficient Blood production in bone marrow or disease.

Alzheimer-Nerves cells degenerate and the brain shrink this condition is most common cause of dementia in the elderly.

Arthritis- is a joint inflammation, which causes severe pain stiffness and swelling. Osteoarthirtis is the most common, it occurs when cartilage covering the end of the bone wear off causing bones to rub and grin leading to severe pain.

Angina –Refers to the sudden chest pain, when the heart is not receiving enough blood & oxygen. Angina pain can occurs when physical exertion, emotional stress, exposure to cold or indigestion. *Symptoms:* resemble a heart attack but are mild and alleviate with rest or nitroglycerin.

Arteriosclerosis- when the artery becomes hard, thick and lose elasticity, it usually caused by diseases, cholesterol or calcium deposits. This condition force blood to travel threw a narrow passageway causing Increase in blood pressure.

Ateriosclerosis-Plaque *(fat)* built up in the artery walls causing narrowing of passageway. This condition may increase blood pressure.

Aneurysm-Is an abnormal dilatation of blood vessels due to disease or weakening of the walls.

Bronchiolitis- It an acute viral infection that affect the smallest branches in the lungs, most common in children under the age of 2, Symptoms may resemble asthma *e.g.* coughing, Fever, wheezing and rales.

CHF- *(congestive heart failure)* - when the heart it unable to pump blood efficiently, leading to *(Congestion)* fluid buildup in the lungs, the body or both, most common on patients with history of MI, hypertension or arrhythmias such as *(Bradycardia)*.

Glossary of Disease & conditions:

Conjunctivitis- (*Pink eye*) it an eye infection highly contagious caused by germs, allergies, or irritant. *Example:* (smoke, or dust). It spread by air or direct touch. Most common Symptoms include: itching, burning red eyes, crusty sticky eyelashes, and drainage from the eyes.

Constipation- the difficult passing of hard, dry feces, common causes include lack of fiber, lack of regular bowel movement and water. Other causes of constipation can be due to various medical complications an example: Cancer and Diverticular disease. If condition persists seek medical advice especially when blood is present.

Croup- a viral infection that causes inflammation of the larynx, trachea and bronchi. It transmitted airborne by a (*coughs or sneezed*) or direct contact with body fluids. Typical in children fewer than 4 years often attack at night and usually follow a cold. *Symptoms:* Fever, a seal bark cough, and respiratory difficulties. It can also aggravate other Respiratory disorders such as Asthma.

Cyst- a sac of fluid or semisolid mass under the skin.

Diarrhea- Watery, lose, frequent stool, common in children. Persistent diarrhea can lead to dehydration and shock. Most common Causes: Intestinal disorders *(VIRUS)*, Overeating, and Indigestion, others causes can be attributing to medical complications seek evaluation especially when blood is present.

Dizziness- *(vertigo) is* a sensation of unsteadiness and lightheadedness, it usually accompanied by nausea, vomiting sweating, or fainting. It caused by a momentary fall in blood pressure. Dizziness can also occur in Stress, fever, anemia and tiredness. If condition persists without cause seek medical evaluation

Epiglottis- A bacterial infection, true emergency that lead to respiratory distress because it produce swelling to the epiglottis which is the cartilage that covers the entrance into the lungs causing airway obstruction.

Epistaxis- is a nosebleed cause by rupture blood vessels or a sign of an internal bleeding due to trauma.

Fainting Temporary loss of consciousness (*Syncope)* most fainting occurs as a result of decreased blood flow to the brain. Causes can be medical as in Hypoglycemia (*Low sugar*) or over stimulation as in fright, drugs, anxiety or fatigue. Persistent fainting without cause must be evaluated.

Gastritis- Inflammations of the Stomach causes may be: virus, overeating, irritants, and alcohol.

Glossary of Disease & conditions:

GERD- (*Gastro esophageal reflux disease*) - or heartburn occurs when stomach acids and juices backup into the throat. Most often caused is overeating, or by a Medical condition where the sphincter does not close tightly enough to prevent acid from escaping. *Caution:* any persistent heartburn must be evaluated especially if accompanied by chest pain.

Hepatitis- An infection that causes liver Inflammation and Jaundice, it transmitted by contact (*blood, stool*) and airborne (*sneezed or coughs*). Most common symptoms includes: yellow skin and white in the eyes, dark urine, abdominal pain, nausea, low grade fever, fatigue and loss of appetite.

Pericarditis- Inflammation of the Pericardium, it's the membrane that enclosed and protects the heart. Causes included certain bacterial, viral , fungi and infections. Others causes include: Myocardial infarction, cancer in the lungs or breast, heart surgery and trauma. Most common signs & symptoms include: Fever and chest pain.

Pneumonia -is an acute bacterial infection of the lungs, it often affect the alveoli tiny air sacs, where gases are exchanged causing difficult breathing.
Most Common signs & Symptoms:

- High Fever, Cough with yellow sputum
- Difficult breathing, possible chest pain
- Chest tightness, possible wheezing

Pneumothorax- when Air enters the lungs often caused by of trauma.

Pneumohemothorax- Air and blood enter the pleural space of the lungs, most often caused by injuries to the lung as in trauma such as stabbing.

Shock- is decreased   body fluids volume as result lack of oxygen and nourishment for the tissues and organs. Shock can lead to dehydration of organs and death. Stages of shock I-compensated shock- when the body tries to compensated, it increases heart rate and strength of contractions, pulse, then increases peripherals vascular resistance. Stage II-Decompensate shock is when the body is no longer able to maintain systolic pressure. Shock is caused by several reason for example: Hemorrhage, infections, trauma, poisoning, heart attack, dehydrations and drug reaction.

Example and Type of shocks:

- Anaphylactic- causes by allergic reaction *e.g.* bee sting
- Cardiogenic- Heart fail to perform
- Hypovolemic- Abnormal loss of body fluids e.g dehydration or blood loss *E.g.* Hemorrhagic.
- Psychogenic- A nervous system reaction e.g. Fainting
- Septic shock-cause by severe infection(*toxins-poisons*)

Emergency assessment

Mnemonics -Is a memory method that uses association for remembering information, below are some most often formula use to assess medical Emergency and patient care.

AVPU *Assess Level of consciousness*

A	Alert & oriented
V	Verbal stimuli
P	Painful stimuli
U	Unresponsive

History Assessment

S	Signs & symptoms
A	Allergies
M	Medications
P	Past medical history
L	Last Meal
E	Events

Status Assessment

C	Critical
U	Unstable
P	Potential Unstable
S	Stable

Pain Assessment

P	Provocation: what caused it
Q	Quality: what does feel
R	Referral: where does it go
R	Recurrence: did it happen before
R	Relief:
R	Region: where does it hurt
S	Severity: rate pain (1-10)
T	Time: when did it began

Chocking

Heimlich maneuver- is a method of abdominal thrust, developed by Dr.Henry Heimlich. This technique will force air from the lungs upward clearing any obstructive object in the respiratory tract. Standing behind victim, place one fist on the midline of body, between waist and rib cage, *(above navel)*. Grab this fist and rapidly deliver 5 inward and upward thrusts. Repeat until object is out or unconsciousness then laid victim on the ground and continue straddle on the side until object is dislodge or emergency arrives. If object is out check for pulse, No pulse begin **CPR**, if pulse is available but no Respiration begin rescue breathing without compressions. *Caution:* Never use abdominal method on infant or female in late pregnancy, instead used the Chest thrust method, it's applied in the same manner as in CPR, and this method is also recommended for obese patients.

	Adult 8 yrs and up	Child 1-8	Infant 0 –1 yrs
Conscious	Check responsiveness Asked Are you chocking? If yes, give 5 quick and upward Abdominal thrust.	Check responsiveness Asked Are you chocking? If yes, give 5 quick Inward and upward abdominal thrust	5 Back blows & 5 Chest thrust
If witness unconsciousness	* Open airway * Finger sweep for object * Give 2 breath *Look & listen for breath to enter lungs causing chest to rise and fall, if breath don't enter reposition head and try again, if unsuccessful* * Give 5 Thrust * Repeats steps until objects dislodged or emergency arrives	* Open airway * Remove object If visible. Do Not use Finger sweeps Method *Finger sweep is when you sweep across cheek with finger for objects, this method not recommended for children's.* * Give 2 initial breath If breath don't enter lungs * Give 5 thrust * Repeats steps until object is dislodged	* Open airway * Removed if visible object. * Ventilate. *Look listen for breath sound and chest rise* * Back blow & Chest thrust * Repeats steps until objects dislodged or emergency arrives

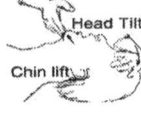

Head Tilt

Chin lift

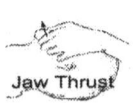

Jaw Thrust

Note: *Proper head position assures an open airway and prevents further injuries. Two method of head position are recommended: Standard Head tilt chin lift or Jaw thrust which moves the jaw only upward, used when suspected spinal or head injuries.*

Facts: *The tongue it's the most common cause of obstruction in an unconscious child's airway.*

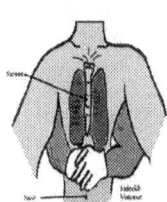

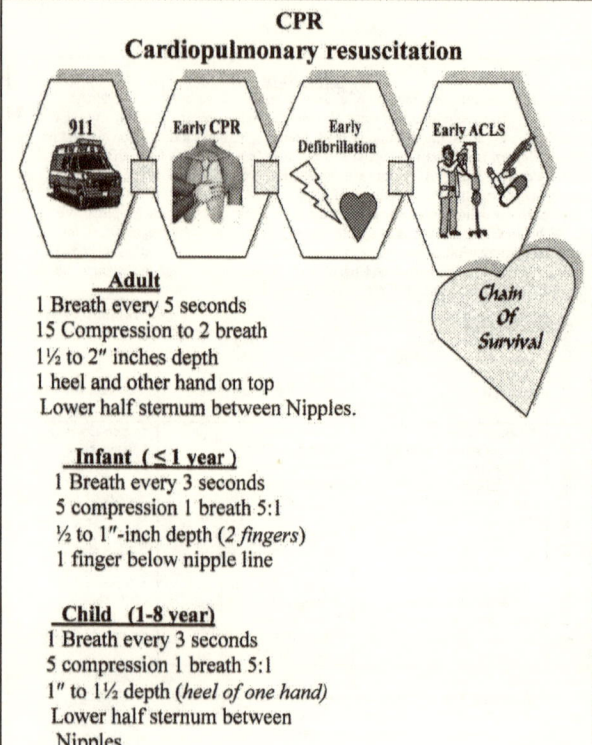

CPR
Cardiopulmonary resuscitation

911   Early CPR   Early Defibrillation   Early ACLS

Chain Of Survival

Adult
1 Breath every 5 seconds
15 Compression to 2 breath
1½ to 2" inches depth
1 heel and other hand on top
Lower half sternum between Nipples.

Infant (≤ 1 year)
1 Breath every 3 seconds
5 compression 1 breath 5:1
½ to 1"-inch depth (*2 fingers*)
1 finger below nipple line

Child (1-8 year)
1 Breath every 3 seconds
5 compression 1 breath 5:1
1" to 1½ depth (*heel of one hand*)
Lower half sternum between
Nipples.

CPR site

NO PULSE BEGIN CPR

Note: *Early defibrillation can prevent death, an AED automatic external defibrillation is used for cardiac arrest, is recommended for adult and a child's older than > 8 years.*
Clinical Death- *occurs when respiration & Heart stop.*
Biological death *-occurs when brain cells die 7-10 minutes, the damage becomes irreversible.*

Oxygen Management

Device	Flow Rate LPM-litters per minutes	% Oxygen Delivers
Nasal Cannula Delivers low concentration of oxygen via the nostrils, it's recommended for COPD patients.	1-6 LPM	24-44%
Simple facemask delivers moderate oxygen. It may be used for minor trauma.	6 7-8 10	40% 50% 60%
Nonrebreather mask delivers High concentration oxygen, Choice for shock, & hypoxia	12- 15 LPM	80-95%
BVM Mask / No Oxygen	Room air	21%
BVM Bag-valve Mask, this method force air into lungs, it has a bag with a reserved oxygen that when squeeze it delivers 100 % of 02.	10-15	80-100%

Pulse Oxymeter

Normal	95-99%	Good
Mild Hypoxia	91-94%	Oxygen
Moderate Hypoxia	86-90%	Oxygen
Severe Hypoxia	< 85%	Emergency care

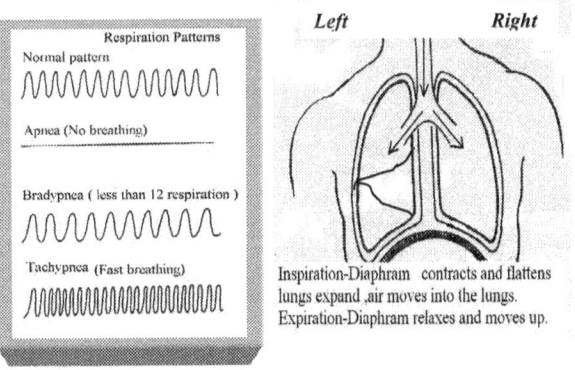

Respiration Patterns

Normal pattern

Apnea (No breathing)

Bradypnea (less than 12 respiration)

Tachypnea (Fast breathing)

Left   **Right**

Inspiration-Diaphram   contracts and flattens lungs expand ,air moves into the lungs.
Expiration-Diaphram relaxes and moves up.

Most Common Medical Abbreviations:

Abd	Abdomen	**Fx**	Fracture
ABG	Arterial Blood Gas	**GERD**	Gastroesophageal reflux disease (*Heartburn*)
AIDS	Acquired immune deficiency syndrome	**GU**	Genitourinary
AMS	Alter mental status	**HTN**	Hypertension (*High Blood pressure*)
ASHD	Arteriosclerosis heart disease	**Hx**	History
a.c.	Before meals	**IDDM**	Insulin dependent diabetes mellitus
b.i.d	Twice a Day	**IM**	Intramuscular (*in the muscle*)
BP	Blood pressure	**IV**	Intravenous (*in Vein*)
BPH	Benign prostatic hypertrophy	**MI**	Myocardial Infarction (*Heart attack*)
Bx	Biopsy	**NPO**	Nothing by mouth
CA	Carcinoma (*cancer*)	**NTG**	Nitroglycerin (Vasodilator-*Dilates arteries*)
CAD	Coronary artery disease	**OS**	Left eye / **OD**- Right eye
CHF	Congestive heart failure	**OD**	Overdose
COPD	Chronic obstructive pulmonary disease	**PID**	Pelvic Inflammatory disease
CVA	Cerebrovascular accident *(Stroke)*	**p.o.**	By mouth *(oral)*
CSF	Cerebrospinal fluid	**PUD**	Peptic Ulcer disease
D/c	Discontinue	**PCN**	Penicillin
DKA	Diabetic ketoacidosis	**q.i.d**	Four times a day
DNR	Do not resuscitate	**RBC**	Red blood cell
DVT	Deep vein Thrombosis	**RHD**	Rheumatic heart disease
DX	Diagnosis	**RUQ**	Right upper quadrant
ESRD	End stage renal disease	**RLQ**	Right Lower quadrant
FBS	Fasting blood sugar	**SIDS**	Sudden infant death syndrome
		SOB	Shortness of breath

Most Common Medical Abbreviations:

S/S	Signs & symptoms	**Ca+**	Calcium
TB	Tuberculosis *(Type of lung disease)*	**Fe**	Iron
TIA	Transient ischemic attack *(mini stroke)*	**Hg**	Mercury
TSH	Thyroid stimulating hormone	**K+**	Potassium
TID	Three times a day	**Mg+**	Magnesium sulfate
TX	Treatment	**NaCl**	Sodium chloride
UA	Urinalysis	**Na+**	Sodium
URI	Upper respiratory infection	**02**	Oxygen *(Clear, odorless gas)*
UTI	Urinary tract infection	**C02**	Carbon Dioxide
VD	Venereal disease		
WBC	White blood cell		
TSH	Thyroid stimulating hormone		
ā	Before		
c̄	With		
s̄	Without		
↓	Decrease		
↑	Increase		
≥	Greater than		
≤	Less than		
−	Negative		
+	Positive		
♂	Male		
♀	Female		

Measurement & equivalents

1 Tbsp = 3 tsp = 16 ml
1 tsp = 5 ml
1 Cup = 8 oz = 16 tsp = 240 ml
1 Lb= 16 oz
1 gal = 4 quart = 3840 ml or 5 L
1 quart = 2 Pint = 960 ml
1 Pint = 2 Cups = 480 ml

Weight:
1 Kilogram (Kg/kg) = 1000 Grams
1 Gram (Gm/gm/ g/g) = 1000 Milligrams (mcg)
1 Milligram (mg)= 1000 micrograms (mcg)

Colors		Greeting	
Red	Rojo	Hello	Holla
Blue	Azul	Goodbye	Adios
White	Blanco	Good morning	Buenos dias
Black	Negro	Goodnight	Buenas noche
Gold	Oro	Please	Porfavor
Yellow	Amarillo	Thank you	Gracias
Violet	Violeta	Sorry	Perdona
Green	Verde	Later	despues

Alphabet

English				Spanish	
A	A	J	Jota	S	Ese
B	Be	K	Ka	T	Te
C	Ce	L	Ele	U	U
D	De	M	Emme	V	Ve
E	E	N	Ene	X	Equis
F	Efe	O	O	Y	I qriega
G	Ge	P	Pe	Z	Zeta
H	Hache	Q	Cu		
I	i	R	ere		

Numbers

One	1	U-no	Thirty	30	Tre-in-ta
Two	2	Dos	Forty	40	Cua-ren-ta
Three	3	Tres	Fifty	50	Cin-cu-en-ta
Four	4	Cua-tro	Sixty	60	Se-sen-ta
Five	5	Cin-co	Seventy	70	Se-ten-ta
Six	6	Se-is	Eighty	80	Ochen-ta
Seven	7	Sie-te	Ninety	90	No-venta
Eight	8	Ocho	When combining numbers used "y"		
Nine	9	Nu-e-ve	to connect, sound like "E"		
Ten	10	Di-ez	Example: 42 = Cuarenta Y Dos		
Twenty	20	Vei-nte	93= Noventa Y Tres		

Body Parts/ Partes del cuelpo

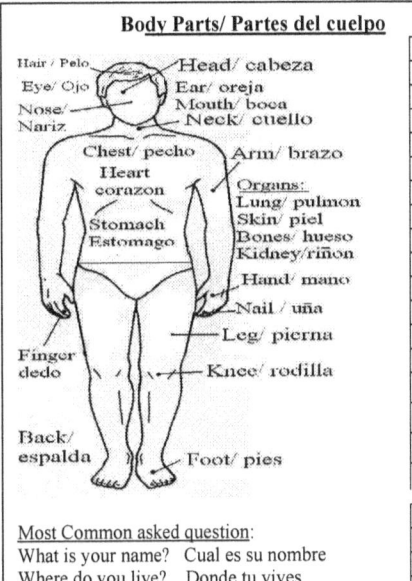

Hair / Pelo
Head/ cabeza
Eye/ Ojo
Ear/ oreja
Nose/
Mouth/ boca
Nariz
Neck/ cuello
Chest/ pecho — Arm/ brazo
Heart
corazon
Organs:
Lung/ pulmon
Stomach
Skin/ piel
Estomago
Bones/ hueso
Kidney/riñon
Hand/ mano
Nail / uña
Leg/ pierna
Finger
dedo
Knee/ rodilla
Back/
espalda
Foot/ pies

up	arriba
down	abajo
Here	aqui
There	alla
More	mas
Less	poco
Happy	alegre
What	Que
Sad	triste
Cry	llorar
Bad	mal
Good	Bueno
Old	viejo
New	nuevo
Yes	si
Now	ahora
Slow	Suave
Fast	Rapido

I	Yo
You	Tu
He	El
She	Ella
They	Ellos
We	nosotros
Why	Porque
What	Que
Where	Donde
When	Cuando
How	Como
Boy	Niño
Girl	Niña
Men	Hombre
Women	Mujer

Most Common asked question:

What is your name?	Cual es su nombre
Where do you live?	Donde tu vives
Where you going?	Donde tu vas
How old are you?	Cuantos años tienes
Do you need help?	Tu necesita Ayuda
What time is it?	Que hora tienes
Where is the pain?	Donde tienes dolor
What Happen?	Que paso
What this?	Que es esto
Come Here?	Ven aqui
Sit down here?	Sientate aqui
Are you tired?	Esta Cansado
Are you Hungry?	Tu tienes Hambre
Do you want to eat?	Tu quieres comer

About the Author

As a child I was always fascinated by the human body. As I got older I became an EMT because I wanted to help others. I work with 911 Emergency Medical Services and responded to varies type of emergencies. Such as heart attack, stroke and even accident. The experience I gained was amazing but I wanted to do more for those in need. I became a medical assistant where I work with one-to-one patient alongside doctors and nurses.

www.ingramcontent.com/pod-product-compliance
Lightning Source LLC
Chambersburg PA
CBHW020335290526
45785CB00005B/2021